4 $\frac{1}{2}$ STEPS

SURVIVING THE RECKLESS ROLLER COASTER RIDE TO RECOVERY

by RANDY WAGNER

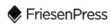 FriesenPress

One Printers Way
Altona, MB R0G 0B0
Canada

www.friesenpress.com

ISBN
978-1-03-914897-0 (Hardcover)
978-1-03-914896-3 (Paperback)
978-1-03-914898-7 (eBook)

1. BIOGRAPHY & AUTOBIOGRAPHY, PERSONAL MEMOIRS

Distributed to the trade by The Ingram Book Company

This is for my parents, who allowed me to live my new life, and for Jake and Alicia in perpetuity, who taught me what's important in a life well-lived life, and for all the friends that never gave up on me. Cheers forever.

CHAPTER ONE

STUPIDITY: THIS SHOULD BE A STEP, BUT IT ISN'T

SOME PEOPLE KNOW WHAT THEY want to be when they grow up. Some become firefighters or cops like it's in their DNA. Others get through high school and still emerge clueless, like a lump of raw clay, unmolded, their future undecided, waiting for their big break around every corner. That about sums me up. I tried to avoid the whole process by not growing up. Instead, I valiantly tried to outrun responsibility.

Thinking back, high school can quickly sort out the rocket scientists from the journeymen. Parents can play a part; they can guide you in a direction *they* approve of, or perhaps you try to realize your potential in college or university, taking course after course until you decide your endgame. You could have one of those weird epiphanies that changes your life and steers you toward your goal. Unfortunately, I had none of these.

So, after two years at Douglas College and one year at the University of Victoria, I hit the ground running at twenty-eight, with zero direction. What was I good at that separated me from the pack? What was my untapped talent? We should all ask ourselves that question. Unfortunately, I never found an easy answer. So after ruling out construction laborer, radio disc-jockey, bouncer, bartender, journalist, municipal worker, Zamboni driver, and Keg waiter, I chose to follow someone else's dream, which is why I find myself sitting in the cheap seats in Theatre Calgary watching *Les Misérables*.

The men dressed casually; some with jeans, some with cotton dress pants, some with T-shirts, and some, like me, are going the extra mile by breaking out the ties and sport coats. Men in the cheap seats don't own tuxedos; they own ties and sport coats. I still wonder why they call it a "sport" coat, because I cannot think of a sport that you could participate in while dressed in the silly thing.

These men joining me in the cheap seats also look bored. They are gazing around, resigned to their fate. I nod at them when we make eye contact. I'm betting every man jack one of them would probably give their little finger to see a beer vendor magically appear at this very moment. I know I would. The women are different, not bored or trying very hard not to appear that way, and they are very aware of their appearance. No "sports" attire for them. Before this significant event, they went shopping. This outing is an occasion for them, and their mode of dress reflects their desire to impress. They are all Cinderella for a night. They wear low-cut gowns that are all the rage this year; the more cleavage and skin, the better. Never a bad thing; in my humble estimation, low-cut gowns should never go out of style.

"Watch the play," says the woman sitting beside me, who knows full well that I would rather be sitting on the fifty-yard line at a football game than at Theatre Calgary. The woman beside me may well be my wife, but if she truly loved me, she would recognize my need to remain uncultured. I'm secretly enjoying the experience, but I wish for a cold beer *and* a shot or two of scotch. A hot dog and a bag of peanuts wouldn't hurt either.

And the conclusion is logical. The miserable, downtrodden lot capering and singing on the stage is doomed. It causes me to sigh audibly. I find their indomitable spirits hard to ignore. Yes, sirree, catchy tunes, good story, plenty of cleavages. It should be enough for anybody, but the stage is located roughly one hundred yards away, by my estimation. About one football field away. Okay, not that far, but the location of the stage is a long way from where we sit. I sigh even more audibly; I love winding up my wife.

"Quit squinting, and especially quit sighing. You sound like you're blowing up an air mattress," says my beautiful wife. But of course, my wife, who probably knows I'm making a big show of squinting and sighing and pointing it out, will only spur me to greater heights of much of the same. I am always ready to be cultured, but culture, it seems, does not come cheap.

The play is over. People start shuffling out all around us, but we're in no hurry because our limo will be waiting. We also have a cold beer and a bottle of champagne on ice waiting for us, and we plan to drive around for a good long while. Drinking and driving around in style will make up for squinting and sighing. We time it right; at least a hundred people are milling about outside the theatre, and it is drizzling, so getting into a limo is a nice luxury. Once settled inside, we cruise Calgary. Cruising takes on new dimensions when one is doing it in a limo, enjoying the luxurious, posh leather interior. We sip champagne and discuss the play like little *Siskel and Eberts* while enjoying the sights of Calgary.

We have not so much picked Calgary as Calgary has chosen us. That's right; our dream is to open a restaurant, a Boston Pizza franchise. The name is a misnomer, as the head office for the franchise is located in Richmond, British Columbia, which is a long way from Boston last time I looked. However, they sell pizza, and the franchise does very well in Alberta. We also have found partners to help fund our little dream. My wife and I could never scare up the down payment for a restaurant. Still, with our new partners, who are initially from Peace River, we are on board as co-restaurant owners due to the strengths of our management potential. My wife's parents took out a second mortgage to get us this far. It is not ideal, but it fast-tracked our way to owning our own restaurant one day.

"To our left here is the Olympic Park . . ." the driver intones with pride. He has given this tour before, and he is obviously still entranced by the beautiful city of Calgary. I can only assume our driver has never been outside of Alberta. "Six lifts, ski jumping, a luge course, and a 400-foot vertical drop," he finishes with a flourish.

"We call those bunny hills one province over," the cynic in me tells him. I'm a province snob. Anyone born in British Columbia is a province snob, and we can't help ourselves.

"Do you have luges and Bobsled runs in your province?" he continues, somewhat piqued.

"Any sport where gravity is your best friend is not what I'd call a real sport," says the cynic, undaunted. Part of me hopes the cynic will wear him down, and then maybe he'll cut the tour short, close the glass partition, and take us to a bar where I can drink in peace. But unfortunately, cruising aimlessly to draw out the limo ride is all part of the process, which quickly loses its luster when we run out of champagne. I am sure doing a lot of whining, especially for someone who is thirty years old and about to own his first restaurant, all because of my wife's parents.

"Wag, will you shut up, enjoy yourself, and quit being such an asshole?" says the woman who is my wife. She calls me "Wag" because it's short for Wagner, now her married name. She also calls me "Wag" because my first name is Randy, and it is not a name I particularly like. It is a unisex name. It means horny in Australia and maybe England, and it's not an excellent chest-thumping guy's name, so I don't think I ever grew into it. "Wag," however, is an acceptable nickname.

"I can't be expected to do both," I tell her. "You can have one or the other. I would gladly stow the comments if we could ditch limo-man and find us a bar without wheels. Anything with a bathroom. Luxury without certain amenities sucks when your back teeth start floating."

Sally and Mike, our partners in excess just for the evening, look at me like I'm nuts. They are the cohorts my wife has chosen to accompany us on our cultural endeavor. Sally and Mike are my wife's close friends. They tolerate me because they like my wife, but they are now offended because I've insulted limo-man and, by association, the entire decadent practice of limo-riding. I give them a look and a shrug that says, "It's your move. What do you want to do?" I have now effectively put the onus on them to decide, although I'm being a bully, and I know it.

If suggestive bullying fails, I'm not above straight out bullying, but intimidation is a last resort, and it never works on the woman who is my wife. She knows this tactic is somewhat of a front. We've only been married for a year or so, but we've more or less been together nine years, on-and-off, and I have no wish nor desire to be a bully in her eyes. But on the other hand, I would not hesitate to bully Mike and Sally in a New York second. They are too concerned with impressing other people, and it's not an endearing personality trait. Primpers and preeners can always benefit from good sound bullying.

"Hey, I know," says Mike, who suddenly has an idea that saves him from future stress. "Why don't we just go back to The Keg, and I'll buy us a couple of drinks? After all, I've got the keys." He holds up the keys he's talking about, and not for the first time that evening. He gives them a good jangling. He jangles his keys a lot because he is a *proud* key jangler, the type of person who feels powerful with many meaningful keys in his hand. He is a primper *and* a preener, but he's also a key jangler. I have to keep reminding myself that my wife thinks the world of these two people, so I flash my best co-conspirator smile and give him an okay nod. If I had my own set of important keys, I would now take this opportunity to jangle them.

"Agreed," I add quickly, post nod because the woman who is my wife is about to suggest something else, and I fear the consequences. She likes getting the feel of a new city, and if I left it up to her, the tour could become interminable. I've seen enough of Calgary and the surrounding area to know that I will not *love* living here, but I might *like* it. I've resigned myself to stoic endurance, but I know I won't live here longer than necessary. I was born in Maple Ridge, in beautiful British Columbia, and I am convinced I will eventually grow old and die somewhere in British Columbia.

"Okay," my wife says reluctantly. She knows she can only push the culture envelope so far, and she knows it's wearing thin. But ultimately, culture makes me thirsty, so heading for The Keg sounds good to me.

Eventually we arrive at The Keg, and it is pretty much closed to the general public, but *we* are not the general public. Mike, the jangler, is the manager of this restaurant. He is the official keeper of the keys, and we can stay as long as we want. He has taken great pains to point this out, and I have taken greater pains to appear suitably impressed because he's buying the drinks.

Before going in, Mike asks, out of the blue, if I would like to see his new golf clubs. It seems a rather silly thing to ask of someone you barely know, but we have discovered that perhaps the only thing we truly have in common is our love of golf—and we are going to have to build from this one commonality—so I comply in the spirit of friendship. It may otherwise be a long night.

We exit the limousine and dismiss the driver after a huge tip, and we all wander toward his car, located at the back of The Keg. The sooner this is over, the sooner I can get my free drinks. He locates the key (more jangling) that opens the trunk of a new Ford Taurus, and he reverently extracts his clubs. It is now my wife's turn to sigh audibly, as she has no interest in golf and considers anyone stupid enough to spend a fine summer day excited about a little white ball is one step above certifiable.

But I am suitably impressed. Although I secretly think that the people who spend the most money on golf clubs are usually the worst golfers, I call his golf clubs a miracle of modern technology, and without much coercing, I "heft" (his word) one of them.

"Go ahead, heft it," he implores me. "Test the weight, give it a good swing," he says. I believe Mike is taking this male bonding thing too far. I am almost willing to buy my own bloody drinks, but politeness rules the day.

"Beautiful," I remark, 'hefting' a five iron like one who knows his golf clubs. I go as far as to find a small patch of grass. Then, after taking out a whacking great beaver tail of a divot on my first practice swing, I say, "Heavy, but firm," like I am indeed a golf club connoisseur, although, for the life of me, I have no clue as to why people get a big woody over golf clubs. "Heavy, but firm," is a conversational gambit that essentially alludes to one thing. Please, just give me a bag that carries twelve beers and an ice pack, and I am good to go. But the divot barely hits the ground before a new idea has formed in my mind.

"You got any smiley-faced, old frog bait balls? You know, spares you could care less about ever seeing again?" I ask. I've momentarily forgotten my free drinks. He looks at me like I'm stunned and he's never heard the term "frog bait."

"I'm referring to balls that have outlived their usefulness unless you're hitting over a giant gully or a body of water you have little hope of clearing. Only Tiger, Jack, Freddy, or Fuzzy would not be caught dead with smiley-faced, frog bait balls in their bags."

"Sort of, but why? There's nothing around here but condos and apartments. You aren't thinking of actually hitting a ball, are you?"

"No way," chirps up the woman who is my wife. She knows how my mind works and immediately realizes that "nothing good can come of this." This is one of my favorite go-to expressions, aptly expressed by a good friend of mine in Maple Ridge. "Nothing good can come of this," is an expression I should have tattooed on my forehead, but I had yet to consider how this night might end.

So I say, "Why not? The chances of hitting a window are so slim that it barely rates a mention. Besides," I'm now expressly addressing Mike, "how will I know what a great set of golf clubs you have here unless I take a good hack at a real live golf ball?" Before my wife can launch further protests, Mike decides that I have brought up a valid point.

"I never thought of that. If you aim away from the apartments and toward that parking lot on the left, what harm can it do? It's way too late for anyone else to be out." So there is hope for Mike yet.

"What harm, indeed," I say. "The nearest building is at least 250-yards away. You would have to give a ball a tremendous whack to get it that far. You'd have to want to hit it that far deliberately. A good solid three wood or a two iron, at least."

"Yeah, okay," says Mike, making up our collective minds.

"Let's get a drink, Sally," says the woman who wishes that at this moment she wasn't my wife, "I'd rather be inside at the bar than out here watching these two idiots, so I can deny that I ever met either one of them when they're hauled off to jail."

Sally dutifully gets the keys and follows disconsolately. I'm not sure whether she understands the whole exchange, so she is better off going into the restaurant. On the other hand, my wife understands what is going on only too well, and she knows she is better off going into the restaurant. No complaints from me, as it allows me to focus my attention on the task at hand.

"A golf ball then, my good man, and a tee," I add, handing back the five iron and getting out of my not-aptly-named sport coat, "and if you would be kind enough to release the big stick, I will give this ball a ride."

"You want a one wood?" he says, unsure about this new wrinkle.

"Sounds good," I say.

"Maybe this isn't such a good idea." You can sense his trepidation.

"Back away then, partner, and give me some room. Your protest shall be duly noted." I know that after liberally imbibing both champagne and beer, my chances of hitting the ball are no better than fifty percent anyway. The consequences of my actions cross my mind only briefly because I am an asshole that rarely considers effects and consequences.

I take a few warm-up swings and find my center of gravity. Not an easy task because my center of gravity is not joining the party. But golf is all about overcoming adversity and incessantly bragging about it afterward. So, I step up to the ball, and I am ready, loose as a goose and raring to go. Warm-up swings are for wimps, anyway. I fully intend to leave nothing in the bag.

I take a deep breath, a moment to find the ball, and then another moment to focus on it. I take an enthusiastic Babe Ruthian hack at it, almost coming out of my Wal-Mart dress shoes. The swing carries right through the ball. I hit it right on the sweet spot of this new-fangled aluminum club, and my ball takes off like a scalded dog.

I have launched this ball beyond anything I could have hoped for, and adversity has been overcome. It is a result I view with pride, while beside me, Mike makes a slight squeaking sound. The ball has sprouted wings. It flies over the highway without so much as a how-do-you-do. It is a shot I shall boast about later on to anyone willing to listen.

I lose sight of it after it clears the highway. I believe it is still rising when it chunks off the aluminum siding of the apartment building across the road. It is a solid chunk sound that I'm sure has just left a crater in the aluminum siding. I feel good about my club selection.

"You fucking idiot. Are you nuts?" says Mike, realizing too late that this may be the case. He has suddenly remembered that he is the restaurant manager right where I have seen fit to tee off. "Jesus fucking Christ, that could have easily gone through a window or a patio door," he continues until I hold out my hand for another ball.

"One more time," I say, and when he stands there stupefied, I am forced to dig a ball out of his bag and tee it up for round two. Mike is now feeling somewhat responsible for my actions, but he knows he has lost control of the situation.

"A little quiet on the tee, please," I implore him. But, son of a bitch, I'm drunk. I close my right eye. It's always been the lazy one.

"You're fucking crazy," he says once again, getting the last word in and, unfortunately, giving me too much to think about on the backswing, which is hardly sporting. My shot suffers accordingly. I fire it off the toe, and although the sound of the clubhead meeting the ball is gratifying, the sound is small potatoes compared to the loud metallic thump the ball makes upon meeting the door panel of Mike's new Ford Taurus. Unfortunately, he has parked it far too close to the tee-off area, paying dearly for his mistake. I immediately declare a mulligan. Mike is not amused, but I can't stop laughing like an idiot.

It is a new car, not yet paid for—as I'm led to understand by the resultant tirade—so the pothole-like dent the errant ball leaves in the door is apparently of some concern to Mike. He tells me what he thinks of my golf game in general and, more specifically, how I have conducted myself tonight. It is a heartfelt tirade, and I feel suitably chastised. I am thereby forced to leave the club on the tee box and forfeit my turn entirely. It seems I have been disqualified, and that is Mike's prerogative since he is the official holder of all the keys of both the restaurant and, unfortunately, the Ford Taurus.

I leave singing something about jingling keys, it is on a loop in my brain. I am beyond drunk and, therefore, cannot be held responsible—a thin defense. I try, albeit half-heartedly, to explain to Mike that things always look better in the morning. Still, he is inconsolable, and I eventually leave him kneeling, fingering the massive depression left by a golf ball I had earmarked for far greater things.

CHAPTER TWO

MORE STUPIDITY: STILL NOT A STEP

THE KEG IS STILL CROWDED, even though the parking lot looked almost deserted. Keys were unnecessary. While the cats are away, the mice will play. The Keg is filled with waiters and bartenders who are now off the clock, and it is time to drink. It is a loud, raucous atmosphere, imminently preferable to the quiet solitude of cruising in a limo.

My wife and Sally have entered this arena and have already become the center of attention. They are both striking women, and they merit the attention they receive. Unfortunately, I have to stand back and watch them for a few guarded minutes. Sally is somewhat embarrassed to be the object of such blatant admiration, but my wife thrives under these conditions. She is an accomplished flirt, this woman I have married, and it is something she does without thought. Long ago, I learned to live with it. I trust her, and I've seen it before, so watching her perform her magic doesn't make me jealous. Still, it does make me wonder—and not for the first time—why she settled for me when there were so many other eligible bachelors out there for the taking, better-looking ones, to be sure. I don't mean to denigrate myself, but in my estimation, I have a character face and an attitude that would sometimes push even the most patient of mothers and wives. But some things are better left unexplained and unanalyzed.

I'm trying not to think about this as I come up behind her as she sits at the bar, and I nuzzle her neck and give her a quick kiss on the cheek. She allows this, but she favors me with a look that lets me know that she is aware, and not entirely thrilled, that I have been outside firing golf balls at the neighbors. I can see she is willing to forgive me so long as nobody was hurt, but I will hear about this incident again, probably in the morning after I have had a chance to think about it. I know all of this because I can read a lot into one of her looks. Despite her reserve, she has taken it upon herself to purchase me a glass of scotch without ice and a cold beer. A promising sign. I have been forgiven for my sins for the time being, so I decide not to tell her about Mike's car yet because I'm sure she'll hear about it later.

"Where's Mike?" she asks.

I cannot lie. "Mike's car sustained a dent in the parking lot. He'll be in soon," I explain rather vaguely. Fortunately, she doesn't push for details.

"Did you enjoy the play tonight?" she asks, changing the subject and leaving me behind a little, but I am used to playing drunk catch up. I still hesitate to answer because it is a tricky question. She already intuits that I enjoyed it, but she is usually too polite to gloat. Her goal to culture me is succeeding, but the continued success of this thankless venture depends on her ability to be humble while I fight the change and make progress on my own time.

"It was okay," I say, shrugging.

"Just okay?" she says.

"It was better than okay. If you and I were all alone in the theatre, I would have wept openly."

"You are so full of shit. You would have rather been at a football or hockey game, but I'm glad we went."

"Me too," I say, and I am glad. I'm pleased to be introduced to these *new* things despite my protestations. My wife knows I can be open-minded and patient when she cons me to go out to participate in what I often refer to as girlie-boy events like plays, symphonies, and theme parties. But she also knows I wouldn't want to make it a steady diet, so she doesn't push.

"When do you want to go back?" she asks me, referring to the impending drive back to where we are staying in Lethbridge. It is two hours away from Calgary—two hours away—and some socializing remains to be done. Ideally, I'd like to skip going to Lethbridge entirely and stay in Airdrie in the tiny apartment we have rented. But we are currently working at another Boston Pizza in Lethbridge. While we are waiting for our restaurant to be built, we have found employment at this restaurant because we know the owners, and they have hired us, so we can fill in our time cards until our restaurant is up and running. They are good people, easy to work for, and the extra training is beneficial for us.

"I'm not sure," I reply. "What are the options?"

"We could spend the night at our apartment and go back to Lethbridge in the morning, or we could make the red-eye drive after we pack. I'm leaning toward the sleepover option."

"Figures, but what are the chances of getting you out of a warm bed at six in the blessed a.m. and making it to Lethbridge by eight? It's already getting late."

"About zero," she says, knowing I am asking a rhetorical question. My wife is an Olympic gold medal sleeper. When she is awake, she exists in an aura of sustained energy. It surrounds her and engulfs her. She has that aura more often than not. She can work for fourteen hours straight without a break or a complaint if she is constantly entertained or challenged. She has never been one to stand still and just let things happen to her. However, the downside of mainlining adrenaline is that she requires an equal amount of sleep to balance it all out. In her perfect world, she would be allowed one hour of uninterrupted sleep for every one hour awake.

I am convinced that this is a genetic thing. Besides my wife, I've known many people who can slumber away an entire day, awake refreshed, and not feel the slightest tinge of guilt that they have wasted the day. Sleep is not a waste of time to these people, and they seem to derive some innocuous pleasure from being unconscious. On the other hand, I would be happy to do away with sleep entirely. I don't dream much, at least I don't remember dreaming much, and sleep only comes grudgingly after hours of lying in bed rehashing the entire day and singing silly songs in my head.

"I've got to be there in the morning," I say. I have already decided that I'd rather make the interminable, monotonous drive back to Lethbridge tonight, and it's a small matter to convince my wife this is the only viable option. I have to be in Lethbridge by eight, bright-eyed and as bushy-tailed as humanly possible, while she doesn't have to be anywhere in particular until noon the next day. I would much rather wake up in Lethbridge than drive there in the morning with very little to zero sleep and a hangover chasing me all the way home.

It's a bit of a bugger, though. The restaurant in Lethbridge is scheduled to receive guests from the head office in the morning. It is a surprise inspection that is not a surprise, but the restaurant must still be up to Boston Pizza standards. Boston Pizza is giant on rules and promoting uniformity. Ten ounces of cheese on that pizza, four ounces of mushrooms on that one, don't skimp on the shrimp, but keep those food costs down, date and rotate, cook by the book, ad infinitum. I'm learning the lingo as I now partially own one of these restaurants, but I am the unofficial kitchen manager in the fledgling franchise in Lethbridge, and head office must be appeased. I have to be there to make a good impression. I have convinced myself that I am an indispensable cog in the kitchen machine and must be present despite the extra effort and inconvenience. The good people who have hired me and my wife did not have to hire us, and I feel we owe them. I take debts between friends and family very seriously. It is my credo. I suspect the head office types will probably come in, do a cursory inspection, and blast off to the golf course, but that is entirely up to them. I have a job to do, and I am thorough if nothing else.

"What if I drive and you sleep," I say, knowing full well that this will be the case regardless.

"Sounds good. It's one o'clock now, so if we get motivated, we can be on the road in an hour and be in Lethbridge by four or four-thirty."

So, I have a couple of Irish coffees to sober up and then a couple more, and in the end, four booze-filled coffee drinks seem about perfect for the drive ahead of me. We say our goodbyes to Mike and Sally. I am still drunk, but I am now a wide-awake drunk. I remind myself I'm thirty years old and invincible; a thought that still haunts me.

We dawdle at our apartment for far too long. We have rented an apartment in Airdrie, a small town close to Calgary, but far enough away that you can shake off the big city dust and see the foothills in the distance. Eventually, we will permanently move down here to run the restaurant. We don't have much in it, as at the moment we tend to spend most of our time in Lethbridge. Although precious time is expended as we sprawl on the barely broken in king-size fresh-from-the-factory mattress for twenty blissful minutes. We kiss, cuddle, take a stress break and wish that the drive ahead of us wasn't inevitable. We are running behind, but a total disregard for the speed limit and chocolate-covered coffee beans should remedy this minor oversight.

We stop and fortify ourselves with even more cups of straight coffee and a dry bran muffin, which my wife swears by to keep us regular, as if being regular is the key to good health. Of course, everyone knows that moderation is the key to good health. I then decide to take bran muffins out of my diet as I am regular as clockwork, but the coffee is appreciated because I'm more tired than expected. I am sure friggin' caffeine is running through my veins but motivated by time restraints, I remember that I have a job to do and staying awake is paramount.

It is past three o'clock when the lights of Calgary are left in the rear-view mirror, and the world appears to end. It's as if there are no other people on the face of the planet. The road stretches endlessly in front of me, a straight piece of blacktop with nothing but farmland on both sides, nothing to look at but fence lines, and an old, dilapidated barn or two standing ghostly in the light fog and the dark fields. They are like silent, brooding sentinels watching the sleeping cattle, with their bowed roofs and old broken boards. Their usefulness is long forgotten.

By now, my wife is fast asleep, curled up in her seat, the seatbelt under her arm, her head against the windshield, snoring softly. Caffeine does not affect my wife. Once it is time for her to sleep, her body just shuts down, and I know I will be hard-pressed to wake her up when we finally arrive in Lethbridge. I am not disappointed, though. I have made drives like this a hundred times, and I generally like the solitude of the open road, accompanied by loud music.

I especially like to drive late at night. I've made the long drive to Montreal twice by myself, only stopping to sleep on the side of the road both times, and I always get a second wind around three o'clock, but the second wind does not want to kick in so far. I turn up the radio and fiddle with the air vents because I'm close to drifting off a little. I continue like this for another hour and a half. My eyes don't shut exactly, but I'm not paying attention either. The road is tedious, and there is very little to break up the trip. Finally, a small backwoods town called Vulcan whizzes by, and the last chance gas station goes by with it. I slap myself awake and open my window—no more coffee stops, junk food stops, or bathroom breaks. I blink the sleep out of my eyes, shake my head again, and stretch as much as someone over six feet can in a compact Toyota pickup truck. I'll be in Lethbridge in twenty minutes. Twenty long minutes, but I'm sure I can stay awake for twenty more minutes. It should be a cakewalk.

I am invincible, after all.

I catch myself dozing off, though, and I shake myself awake more than once. At least I think I'm awake. What I am is hypnotized. The road rolls by, and I don't even blink. A more competent guy would have packed it in by now and admitted defeat, but I am stubborn. Stubborn trumps smart where I come from, and the truck is on "cruise control" set to fifty-five miles an hour.

In reality, my mind is already fast asleep, and it has sped off into the ether to seek refuge from the monotony of this continuous stretch of blacktop. I'm thinking about the inspection from the head office types. Jim and George may be there, one of them or both. The kingpins of Boston Pizza. I'm already teeing up my ball on the first hole and cracking my first cold one. I am asleep with my eyes open. If I were any more relaxed, I would become part of the bucket seat I'm sitting in, but somewhere in the recesses of my brain, I have convinced myself that I can continue driving even with my eyes closed.

At the time this seems so logical. After all, the truck has made this trip twenty times or more, and by now it requires little or no direction from me. I think that everything will be hunky-dory as long as I wake up now and then and check on the truck's progress. It is on cruise control, after all. At this point (I believe), I close my eyes and fall asleep.

An air horn goes off somewhere far, far away. My subconscious mind hears it, but it filters the sound out, as it doesn't belong in my dream. My dream is all fuzzy and warm, with soft beds and fluffy pillows. It goes off again, though, and I can't ignore it. It has spoiled my dream. I will have to wake up, find the source of the air horn, and make it stop before I can continue sleeping. Again, it doesn't belong in my dream. My gluey eyes come open slowly and reluctantly.

The first thing I see is a white barricade in front of me when my eyes finally focus, and I have only a millisecond to wonder why someone would put up a white fence in the middle of the road. But unfortunately, I have absolutely no time to apply the brakes, and we are through the barrier and going nose-first into a large ditch before I can react.

The next few seconds are entirely filled with sound and fury, crunching metal, breaking glass, excruciating, sharp pain in the back of my neck, and then the relief of total blackness.

CHAPTER THREE

PAIN AND CONFUSION: STILL NOT A STEP

SOMEWHERE, MY WIFE IS SCREAMING. She is worried about the truck. She thinks it will start on fire or explode. Don't be silly. That only happens in bad movies. But she may be right in this case because all I can smell is the overwhelming, cloying stench of gasoline. It surrounds me, and I can taste it in the back of my throat. I should be exiting the truck in due haste, but this will not happen anytime soon because I can't seem to move. It feels like I'm encased in concrete, hovering on the edge of consciousness. Everything is in super slow motion. My arms and legs each weigh a thousand pounds, and I can feel a trickle of something liquid and warm running down the back of my neck. In the dim recesses of my mind, I know that I have fucked up on a significant level. I know this because I can repeatedly hear someone saying, "I've fucked up," in a pathetic monotone with the needle stuck in the groove of a bad record. It takes a while to figure out that I am that someone, and once I figure it out, I make a concerted effort to change the record.

I changed it to, "Someone help my wife. She's hurt. Someone help her." I know she is hurt because I can hear her crying and screaming right in my ear. I want to hold her and tell her everything will be alright, but my eyes will not focus. My head won't turn either. I try to lift my arms again, but something keeps them down. I believe it is the seat belt. It is far too tight, and I can feel it biting into the flesh of my shoulder and neck. It has somehow gotten tangled around my arms; try as I might, I can't lift them. There is pain. Oh, is there ever—the fucking deep, mind-bending pain of red-hot knives sticking into my neck. It is a hundred times worse than any headache I've ever experienced. There are fireworks behind my eyes; I can almost hear my teeth cracking. I am gritting them so hard it hurts my ears. My entire face is squinting with pain, confusion, and a sense of panic. Mercifully, I black out again with my head lying limply on the steering wheel. My last thought is that the steering wheel is in the wrong place. It seems far too close to me.

When I struggle back to consciousness, my wife is right beside me. I don't know how long I've been out cold, but my wife has stopped crying, and now she's talking to me, but she's talking way too loud and way too fast. Her words are rushed and strung together, and it suddenly occurs to me that she's on the wrong side of the truck. She should be on the right side, not the left side. How could she get on the left side of the truck? As near as I can recall, I am the one driving and she is a passenger, not the other way around. I black out again for another minute or two while I ponder this new development.

I know I've passed out briefly because I don't remember the door of the truck opening, yet someone is trying to pull me out of my seat. However, there is no way they will budge me because my seat belt is too tight. I understand my wife is trying to get me out of the truck because she is still concerned about the damn thing starting on fire, evident by the panic in her voice and the violent way she is tugging on my body. I want to reassure her that cars—and in this case, small trucks—don't spontaneously combust. While she's at it, could she please untangle me from the constricting seat belt holding my arms down at my sides? But I can only make croaking sounds, and I still repeatedly say "I fucked up" in a small voice. It is hard to get a breath. It feels like someone huge and heavy is sitting on my chest.

Then there is a sudden sensation of movement. My seat belt has finally been disengaged, although I do not recall how or when. I'm being pulled from the truck, removed bodily from the truck, and dragged along the ground, but the strange thing is that I can't feel the earth under my feet. So I've decided that my legs must be numb, maybe broken, but I believe a slight pull on my ankles will line everything up.

All this is occurring, and I am distant from it, like I'm there, but not *really* there. My eyes still stubbornly refuse to open. It is the weirdest thing. I am conscious but not enough to help myself, and the smell of gas is still overwhelming.

I know it's my wife pulling me through the haze because she can't stop reassuring me that everything will be all right. I want to ask my wife what is wrong with my legs, but we stop moving, and I feel the back of my head hit the earth. It is the last thing I remember.

CHAPTER FOUR

TOTAL CONFUSION: STILL NOT A STEP

WHEN I FINALLY WAKE UP, I am in motion again, only this time I'm in another vehicle, and I'm not the one doing the driving. I can hear the sound of wheels on the pavement, I can feel every pothole. There is an antiseptic smell—a smell I remember from the times I found myself in the Maple Ridge emergency ward in my younger days, a place I had been far too often in my life. I'll never forget this smell, as it equates with a sense of pain and suffering, stitches late at night, or a broken nose being reset and stuffed with cotton. I want to ask someone about the smell, but I'm still unable to open my eyes, and it still feels like an immense, heavy person is sitting on my chest.

I've lost track of how many times I've passed out and woken up again. We are no longer in motion. The only thing spinning is my head. I'm awake this time because I can hear a drill in the distance. It is an unmistakable sound that doesn't seem to fit in with the situation; it is out of place. Why would someone start up a power tool in a moving vehicle? Am I still in a moving vehicle? Again, it doesn't feel like it, but when did I get out of it?

Now, this part is sketchy. When I look back on the accident, there is a definite time sequence to the whole affair, but it all jumbles into one big fucking mess. I make a concerted effort to concentrate on the sound of the drill. The sound becomes more apparent and more defined. It is almost as if the power drill was right before my eyes or just above them. I'm confident I would see the drill if I could open my eyes, but my eyes stay cemented shut no matter how hard I try to open them. I feel pressure on my forehead above my right eye, the pressure of being restrained, and a new sort of pain. Someone *is* attempting to drill into my skull! But that thought is ludicrous. I must be mistaken, as what right-minded individual would drill into another man's skull?

I decide to leave my body to get a better look, and I'm now standing beside myself. I was never a great believer in out-of-body experiences, and I am not remotely religious, but it seems so clear in my mind like I'm watching it. A guy in a white shirt is taking core samples of my brain. He's already finished drilling two exploratory holes in my forehead. He's now going around to the back of my skull.

I can hear him, and he sounds defeated. "What a mess, this guy needs stitches real bad," he says, and then I'm back in my body, and I'm convinced that I imagined the whole thing. It's a messed up, horrible dream, but I realize something is wrong. Big-time wrong, as I still can't feel my body; it will not respond. It just feels too heavy to lift. Or it's restrained somehow, but I can't *feel* the restraints. I should feel something, the bite of handcuffs or someone holding me down. A situation I have been in way too many times.

I am still trying in vain to wake myself up because I don't want to be here anymore. The pain has returned, and it is intense. It squeezes my shoulders and my neck and makes my jaw clench. All I want to do is take a deep breath, but I can barely breathe. I'm sucking in tiny breaths one at a time. A steady pulse is banging inside my head as if my skull is too small to contain my expanding brain. Maybe that's why they are drilling holes. They are trying to let out a part of my brain. It's going to ooze out to release the pressure inside my skull. I can hear the drill's sound when it hits the bone in the back of my head; it bites slightly, and I think I can feel my hair being pulled. I imagine all the hair on my head wrapping itself around the drill bit. It is a blessing when I pass out once again.

CHAPTER FIVE

THE FIRST STEP, THE BIG ONE: DENIAL

IT'S DARK NOW, DARK AND deathly quiet. I am in a morgue. My head has cleared somewhat, and I know I've been in a car accident, but that seems like a lifetime ago. In the meantime, it feels like I have been buried alive up to my neck because my limbs will still not respond, and I can't seem to get enough air into my lungs.

I know my eyes are partially open because I'm blinking, but nothing is coming into focus. I wonder if I am dead. Since I have no experience with being dead, this seems like a good possibility. I close my eyes and open them several times to clear away the gluey crud that built up around their edges. My efforts are rewarded, and finally I see the light. It's more of a lack of complete darkness than light. A hazy, gray light is coming from a door that someone has left open; it's kind of a soft fluorescent glow from far away, like a beacon at the end of a long, dark hallway. If I'm dead, this light should be brighter, and by all accounts I should be traveling towards it. I try to turn my head to see where the light originates, but this creates a world-ending, punching ache behind my eyes. The hurt picks up momentum. It grows into an all-over pain in my head and neck as if my head is on fire, and I'm gritting my teeth so hard I can feel it from my jawline to my ears again. I'm chomping down and grinding my molars together, creating a loud buzz in my ears as I wait for them to splinter and crack from the sustained pressure. An involuntary groan escapes between my parched lips, and I must close my eyes again. I close my half-open eyes, try to swallow, and remember how the hell I got here in the first place.

I vaguely recall someone drilling holes in my head. This can't be true, but it must have happened because there are white-hot points of localized pain right above both eyes and in the back of my skull, right where I'm sure I heard or *saw* them drilling. The pain doesn't end there. It continues down the back of my head and into my neck. It stops right above the point where my shoulder blades come together.

This new pain between my shoulders wins the overall contest, raging in the upper extremities of my body. It feels like an enormous weight tugging on my skull, and the only reason my head hasn't popped right off my shoulders is that the bones and muscles at the back of my neck hold it there, but they are slowly losing the battle. I try to move my head to relieve the insistent, unrelenting drag, but it ramps the pain up to a new level. I moan again, slightly louder this time. Maybe if I could just lift my hands to my head, I could relieve the persistent tugging sensation and keep my skull from popping right off my shoulders, but my hands are tied down. They refuse to respond. I wonder why my hands would be tied down. If I could only clear the fog, I could figure this out. But unfortunately, if this is what it's like to be dead, it is a highly overrated experience: no *bright* light, no angels, only jagged rivers of hurt traveling up my neck from the shoulders to the top of my head. The rest of my body feels numb, almost like it has ceased to exist.

I am completely and utterly confused, and I can't seem to focus. I know I am crying, as I can feel the tears trickling down my cheek. I try to call out, thinking there has to be someone behind the door with the soft fluorescent light. I want explanations, but when I try to shout, the aching in my neck flares up and all that comes out is a garbled bray. It is a sound a distressed donkey might make. A donkey caught in a leg-hold trap. At least the pain lessens while I ponder this new dilemma.

It is the first clue I have that they have drugged me. My mind is swarming with activity, but it cannot focus on any one thing for more than a second, and my thoughts jumble and bounce around like balled-up socks in a dryer. Then I realize I'm not alone after all. There is someone beside me, someone real skinny. The shadows in the room could easily obscure a person. I can't make him (or her) out clearly because I can't turn my head to get a good look.

"Hey," I croak, but I don't get any response.

"Hey, buddy," I say again, a little louder because I have managed to work some saliva around in my mouth. It seems essential that I still have all my teeth, but I don't know why. Old habit, I suppose. I have made an effort to draw air into my lungs, but they reject the idea that oxygen is essentially good for them. So it's time for a new approach.

"Hey, fuckwad, whoever you are, untie my arms and get this fucking contraption off my head. It's killing me. Yeah, I'm talking to you. Who the hell else would I be talking to?" I went all *Taxi Driver* on him, but this new approach exhausted me. My mouth is bone dry, and I decide to just give up and go back to sleep. Sleep sounded pretty darned good right now. The questions about how I got here will just have to wait until I've rested. And then the light is blocked slightly. Finally, someone sticks their head around the doorframe where the light originates.

"He's awake," is all that's said before the head disappears, and I'm alone again. Nobody, it seems, is in any hurry to talk to me. So I take one last shot at the skinny person.

"Look, partner," I say in a hoarse whisper, and even that little effort further exhausts me. "What the hell is wrong with me? My arms and legs don't seem to be working. There's something attached to my skull, and it's playing a game of tug-of-war with my head. It's a game I am not winning."

"He's talking to himself," I hear a female voice say behind the door where the light emanates. I decided that maybe I'll have better luck with whoever was behind the door than I had with the skinny person beside me. But I cannot shake the fog.

"I'm not fucking talking to myself," I say as loud as my scratchy throat will allow, which turns out to be not very loud at all, but it initiates the first actual response I get since I've been awake. No less than three people bustle into my room, and right from the get-go, they're all business. Nobody is smiling.

One says, "Go wake up his wife," and suddenly there are only two people, two ladies by the look of it, ladies in uniform. The second lady starts administering to the skinny son of a bitch that wouldn't talk to me, shaking him—I've decided it's him—and moving him around.

"That guy doesn't say much," I say by way of introduction. It makes the one lady laugh a little. It is painful to speak, like gargling sand.

The other lady is leaning over my bed, adjusting my pillow and fussing with the blankets. "Are you comfortable?" she asks.

"No, my fucking head hurts," I respond without thinking. I'm usually not much for cursing, as it always seems trite and redundant. A wasted exercise unless there's a point to be made, and this point has to be hammered home with a four-letter-or-better word that has shock value. This situation cries out for some good old-fashioned cursing. "My fucking throat is dry, and I can't move my goddamn arms," I finish, confident now that I've stated my concerns adequately.

"You've been in an accident," the lady fiddling with my pillows says. "Your wife will be here shortly—she's fine, by the way—but you, on the other hand, have sustained some damage to your vertebrae."

"My vertebrae, what're vertebrae?" I ask the lady fussing with the pillows, but I've answered it in the back of my mind even as I pose the question. A vertebra is part of the spinal column. The spinal column protects the spinal cord that carries messages to the rest of the body. While digesting this, the accident replays itself in bits and pieces, coming back slowly with fuzzy edges.

I fell asleep—this I remember well—and I vaguely recall hitting a barricade. This last part is a little more than fuzzy, like a nightmare that hangs on the edge of your memory even after you've become fully awake. You're afraid, but you can't quite remember what exactly it is you're so scared of; imaginary monsters or real ones?

Logic dictates that the fussy lady must be a nurse, but what does "sustained some damage to your vertebrae" mean, exactly? Even as I finish this thought, the other lady in uniform brings the skinny guy into focus, and I realize that I have been having a one-sided conversation with an I.V.

pole for the better part of the last ten minutes. Plastic bags filled with fluid adorn the top; it's like looking at a scarecrow with its arm out, and clear plastic tubes snake out of the bags and attach themselves to my wrists.

The whole situation does not bode well. I make a real concerted effort to move my arms and legs for the first time. Nothing happens. I try to curl my fingers and make a fist. Nothing happens.

It's then, at that moment, that it finally dawns on me that my body is not mine anymore. I can't feel the bed underneath me. I was so concerned about my head becoming separated from my shoulders that I didn't realize virtually everything below the significant pain was dead. My toes don't wiggle, and my knees don't bend. For all I know, they aren't even there anymore.

Panic sets in briefly while I recollect stories of people in this position before me, people like Rick Hansen, Stephen Hawking, and a couple of junior hockey players whose names I forget. I also think of the Vietnam Vets who came back from the war depressed, psychological shells of their former selves like the guy in *The Deer Hunter* or Tom Cruise in *Born On The Fourth Of July*. I try harder to move my limbs, determined that I will not be like one of these people.

"What happened to me?" I ask, fearing the answer but unable to stop asking the question. My thoughts are no longer jumbled. Fear is a great motivator for staying awake to fight the drugs they've pumped into me, and I'm trying hard to figure out my predicament.

"You've been in a car accident," the nurse fussing with my pillows explains patiently.

"I know I've been in a goddamn car accident, for Christ's sake. That's not what I asked. I asked, what the fuck happened to me?" I don't want to curse and swear, but I can't seem to stop.

"I'll let the doctor explain," she says. "Your wife should be down here any minute, she can fill you in on some of the details."

With that said, the woman who is my wife enters the room as if on cue. She looks worried. My wife has looked worried before, but she seems distraught this time, a different worry than I have ever seen before. Her eyes are puffy and red, and her hair is disheveled from lying down or sleeping.

4 and ½ Steps

She looks like she just woke up. It is possibly the only time I have seen something akin to pity and distress in my wife's eyes.

"Hi Wag," she says softly as if I'm made of crystal and any loud noise might shatter me into a million pieces. "Something is rotten in the state of Denmark"—or in this case, Lethbridge—and I want to get to the bottom of it.

"I'm going to ask you some questions now, okay?" I start before she can whisper another word. "And I expect real honest answers here, too—no bullshit." I pause to let the gravity of my request set in before I get started, and then I let it rip with a spate of queries that have been building up since consciousness—absolute consciousness—returned. "I want to know what happened to my arms and legs? How bad is the truck? Did I fall asleep? Where the hell are we anyway, and why do I feel like there are three fucking guys trying to remove my head from my body?" Tears come to her eyes before she starts to speak. Tears are not a reassuring sign.

"Wag, you drove the truck into a ditch," she says, and then the tears come. She can't rein them in any longer. She has answered the only question I could figure out for myself. I am not getting any wiser, but the one answer is enough for now. I'm out of energy. I'm exhausted, and truth be known, all I want to do is go back to sleep. I still want to know the answers to the rest of my questions, but I'm beyond tired like I've been awake for six days and seven nights. I've been in a twelve-round title bout, and I've lost badly. I feel like George Chavalo must have felt after meeting Muhammed Ali, and just like George, I'll wake up with a headache and a sore body. I'll feel even worse on the third day. That's just the way these things play out. I just need to know one more thing before I rest up for the next round.

"Am I paralyzed?" I ask, and damned if I don't drift off before I hear the answer.

CHAPTER SIX

STEPS ONE AND TWO: DENIAL AND SOME ANGER

IT'S MORNING WHEN I WAKE up. At least, I'm under the impression it is morning. The blessed light of day is coming through the windows, and I can finally take in my surroundings. I'm in a primarily white, unadorned (heavy on the plain) twenty square foot room with no pictures, no knick-knacks, no brickbats, no crackerjacks (*Dr. Seuss* is my go-to guy when I'm fucked up), with blinds on the windows and a chart on the far wall. It looks like a chart diagramming the skeletal structure, and there's one beside it showing how blood flows throughout the body. It seems a lot like a road map of a foreign country from a distance, something you would see in a doctor's office. I'm happy, stoned, and overwhelmed by pain, a weird combination. Finally, I fall asleep again, and it is the sleep of the dead.

When I wake up, I feel awful, sick, and sore. "Good morning," I say to the I.V. pole because there is nobody else in the room, and I'm lonely and more than a little scared and fucked up. My throat is raspy, like it's been dragged over one hundred miles of dunes, and I sound like I've been gargling with cheap booze and cigarettes my whole life. I could sing bad country songs about trucks and old dogs.

"So, you want to get me something to drink, my lanky little friend? A dry gin Martini would be nice, with four pickled onions." I try not to cough, but I can't help it. My body spasms as it tries in vain to push air out of my lungs, but when I try harder to cough, the spasms only intensify. The pain lurking in the back of my neck is forcing itself to the forefront. It is a living thing. "Oh, and throw in a glass of water while you're at it; lemon water if you've got it. I'm dying here, and it looks like it's just you and me, partner. Sorry if I was a touch rough on you last night. Finding out that your limbs might not work can be a real bitch."

Even as I'm giving the I.V. pole my drink order and bringing him up-to-date on my life, I'm also trying to flex and bend any extremity that will heed my commands, and I'm having zero luck. My body is insubordinate and mutinous, and there is very little I can do to remedy this situation, especially since every attempt at movement makes my neck hurt that much more. The pain is getting tired of just lurking, and it is on the edge of being full-blown. It wants to yell at me. It does not want to whisper anymore.

But I'm not panicking because I can now see my body spread out in front of me, and as near as I can tell, all the essential parts are present and accounted for as I can see the tops of both feet. I can feel a minor, distant, prickling sensation where the I.V. tube enters the back of my wrist, and I take this as a good sign. Any sensation, even prickly pain, is somehow reassuring.

My fingers will still not curl, and I can't clench my fists. My toes and feet might as well be in a different time zone, and I am nearly exhausted from trying to flip my legs over the side of the bed, but at least I'm whole. Thank goodness for small miracles. It seems strange that I would become weary from just trying to move my body even though none of my exertions have met with any success.

I suddenly realize I'm grinding my teeth with the effort, and the pressure of my molars gnashing together is sending shooting pains into the back of my neck. I want to scream in frustration, but I clench my teeth again, even harder until I'm sure they will crack. My exertions are getting me nowhere in a hurry. I will myself to relax. I take five to six deep breaths, exhaling slowly, closing my eyes, and letting calmness settle over me. It's a calmness I don't feel, but it unclenches my jaw and gives me a chance to gain some perspective—bad air out, good air in, repeat several times. Take another inventory. I'm taking a lot of inventory lately.

As near as I can tell, my body is no longer mine. My control has been hijacked. I'm skirting the edge of panic. I know a little something about the spinal cord, and I have done it some injustice that has rendered my body—a body I'm rather fond of—immobile and motionless from the shoulders down. I can barely turn my head.

I can tell there are pillows under my shoulders and around my neck. I can feel pins and needles in my elbows where my arms are resting on the bed, and I can make my wrist flex imperceptibly, not much, but just enough to let me know it is not my imagination. Beyond that, I am fixed and immovable, encased in concrete. I would probably be in extreme panic mode right now, but I have enough drugs coursing through my system to anesthetize an elephant. Every moment is a sea of fog. I go in and out of consciousness, and the moments of muddled clarity that I do have don't last long.

"If this is it, shoot me now," I say to no one in particular, unsure whether I mean it. It's something people just say when they're in an extreme situation they can't control and pain envelops them, but do they mean it?

Someone on the other side of the door has heard me, and I hear rustling. Water is turned on and off in the mystery bathroom, and a nurse appears around the door. In the light of day, I can tell she is a nurse, the uniform is a standard nurse issue, and she is wearing a nametag. Only supermarket clerks, waitresses, bank tellers, and nurses wear nametags. I immediately rule out the possibility of being in a supermarket, a restaurant, or a bank, so logic dictates that this must be a hospital. All thoughts that this is a bad dream and I'll wake up in my bed have dissipated like the morning mist meeting the noonday sun. It is finally hitting home and becoming clear, the brutal realization that I am indeed paralyzed, and I am not sure how to deal with this. Lashing out is my only option. The nurse is convenient.

"Get me the fuck out of here," I say before I can stop myself. It's silly to ask this of a nurse I've just met. My mind is working in non-concentric circles. My thoughts are wisps that refuse to coalesce into complete rational ideas. I must be drugged, almost insensate, because I'm usually sensible and polite to the point of distraction. So, I try to communicate again with even less desirable results.

"Let me have my brain back, will you. No more goddamned drugs," I'm not precisely sure what I'm asking, but it all makes sense in my fractured troubled state. The next thing I know, I utter up an almost insane chuckle. "Let my people go, untie me goddamnit, and we'll all just get on with our fucking day." I leave it there, relatively confident that we now understand each other. At least the nurse is smiling, but I'm not sure if it's with me or at me.

"You're on Demerol," she says, as if this explains everything. She's behind me, out of my field of vision, playing with something attached to my head. I feel a brief respite from the remorseless tugging.

"Perfect, just don't move," I say, but she isn't listening. So instead, there is more movement behind me.

A shooting, searing wreath of sustained agony jumps into my head, and I hear her say, "Sorry about that," through the steady roar of pain in my head.

"Don't do that again, please, or I will seriously have you so killed," I murmur through my clenched teeth. If this continues, I will grind my teeth down to bloody nubs. The throbbing ache in my head has miraculously cleared up some of the mist. Pain is an excellent benchmark. It brings everything back into focus.

"Okay," she says in such a way that lets me know I'm not being taken seriously at all. "Your wife will be back in shortly. You're on a Heparin drip, and a dose of Demerol is ready to go, but I'll hold off until you've talked to your wife if you like. The doctor will also be in as soon as he finishes next door. In the meantime, is there anything I can do to make you more comfortable?" She says this with genuine concern in her eyes and her voice. Sure, try to kill me one minute, and then offer up a big heaping helping of hospitality shortly afterward.

"Aside from that infernal tugging sensation, unbearable pain from the shoulders on up, and being paralyzed from the shoulders on down, I couldn't be better. Top of the fucking world, Ma. Look, no hands." I barely know what's going to come out of my mouth next. I am not entirely comfortable being the object of so much concern, and I want her to go away, but I know she is only doing her job.

"Look, lady," I add, by way of explanation, "I'm feeling a little fucked over right now. So I want to go back a couple of days and start all over again. But if that isn't possible, I am determined to be miserable, but it has nothing directly to do with you, unless there is a time machine close by and you're keeping me from booking some quality time on it."

"I understand," she says.

"How could you?" I shoot back. "You're not the one fucking paralyzed then, are you?" I'm out of line, and I know this even as I'm snapping at her. I am just friggin' angry, and I feel like I'm getting nowhere fast.

"No, I don't truly understand, but I've been on this ward for six years and I've seen many people recover entirely and walk out of here."

"So what are you saying? Is there a chance I might not be paralyzed for life here or what?" I don't want an absolute answer to this question, and she doesn't disappoint me. She leaves wiggle room.

"I'll let the doctor talk to you."

"Why? What can the doctor tell me that you can't?"

"Be patient, Mr. Wagner," she says cheerily. It's always a bad sign when they call you "Mister."

"I've got a fucking choice? Patience is not my strong suit right now," I say with contrition.

"No, I see that," she answers, and there's that sound of both concern and pity.

"Great, wake me up when I've got a choice. Fill me up with more drugs." Again, I am sarcastic and surly, but she has given me my first small ray of hope. Perhaps this condition I find myself in might not be permanent after all. It's the best news I've heard so far, and I want to give my friend the I.V. pole a big thumbs up, but I can't quite manage it. My hand is still not cooperative, bringing me back to Earth with a thump. I'm going to recover entirely, and I can't even lift my stinking, rotten thumb.

The Demerol plays ping pong with my brain for the next hour, like that Atari game I played for six hours one Christmas. I drift in and out of consciousness. It seems more like days, but there is a clock on the wall, and the hands are moving, albeit very slowly. I think I can distinctly hear the seconds tick away. At some point I notice someone else in the room with me. A young guy dressed up like a doctor, wearing a white lab coat. He's chewing on the end of his glasses, looking at a clipboard. He *is* young, at least much younger than the doctors I'm used to seeing.

"Greetings, stranger," I say, letting him know I'm awake and wishing him no harm. There are clouds on the ceiling that I've never noticed before, or are those water stains?

"Greetings," he says right back at me.

"Are you the man with all the answers?" I ask. "I want to get to the bottom of this mystery."

"What mystery is that?" he asks, and it forces me to blink several times. The clouds dissipate as the ceiling tiles come back into focus.

"The mystery of why I'm unable to move, how I came to be in this state, and when I can get on with the blissful drudgery that was my normal life?"

"Well, I can help you with the first part of the mystery. You came in two days ago with an injury to the cervical spine area, and we are now realigning your vertebrae, pending an operation. I'm Doctor Dumars."

"Finally, someone willing to share some information." I sigh, deeply relieved, and at the same time tentative. So far I've just been guessing, and now that I might hear the whole truth and nothing but the truth, I fear the answers. I remember an old lawyer maxim about never asking a question unless you already know the answer, though this maxim has no place here. "Pending an operation?" I ask, perplexed, "I assume that means I have broken something, and you're assuming you can fix it?"

"Not quite that simple, I'm afraid."

"Fuck me, I knew it. Is this a good news, bad news thing?" I say, suspecting all along that this is indeed the case. He nods slowly, letting me know I'm not entirely off the mark. On the bright side, this is preferable to a straight-on bad news scenario, but barely. "Give me the bad news first."

"The bad news is that you are experiencing some loss of sensation in your lower body—"

"Well, duh, that part is fucking obvious. I no longer want to think about the bad news at the moment." I'm wondering if he understands a word I'm saying. There's a lot of that going around. *I* barely know what I'm saying.

"It may or may not be permanent."

"That's the *good* news. Is that the best you can do?"

"It's way too early to tell. When a spinal cord injury first occurs, there is immediate swelling, which causes a loss of feeling in your extremities."

"So my entire body from the shoulders down is what we are now calling my 'extremities'?"

"Well, in your case . . ."

"Of course, in my case. Who the fuck else would we be talking about here? I'm asking straightforward questions, Doc. Don't patronize me, and don't sugar-coat the whole fucking thing. Now, let's start over. I feel fuck-all from about the neck down, and I only hope this is a temporary setback. I'll run with that if you tell me differently, but this not knowing shit is killing me." I realize I'm yelling at him. He looks momentarily stunned, but he recovers quickly. I know I am also rambling somewhat, striking out again, but the good news contained no great revelations, and the bad news wasn't as good as I was hoping it would be.

"You've got a C-5-6 complete separation of your spinal cord, so we are dealing with this while assessing the permanent damage. Only time will tell the severity of the damage you've suffered, but we are currently trying to stretch the damaged vertebrae so they line up and we can repair them. It may take a week, or it may take longer. I will show you the x-rays if you think you're ready for that, and we do have a mirror available if you wish to look at what we are trying to achieve. Unfortunately, you are immobile at this point, and sometimes, well, most times, people want to look at themselves."

"You bet, I want to see the complicated series of ropes and pulleys attached to my fucking head, and you said 'damaged' way too many times."

"Okay, let's start from the beginning. What you have attached to your head is called a Halo. Have I said that already? It's attached to your head to stretch out the vertebrae until they line up, and then we will have to repair the damage one step at a time. The stirrups on your shoulders align your head, so you will have trouble moving. You will experience some pain if you try."

"Well, isn't that fucking ironic. I'm thinking about all the bad shit I've done in my life to get me to this point, and you guys are attaching a Halo to my skull." I was making lame comments, trying hard to be jocular, but the gravity of what he had told me was not lost on me. I have fucked up big time. Although minor damage goes a long way from what I know about the spinal cord, the fact that I have totaled off some vertebrae makes the prognosis grave. I decide to go for the ten-million-dollar questions early, as the doctor moves around the mirror so I can see the fucking monkey bars attached to my head.

"What's the bottom line, Doc? Am I fucked over for life? Am I going to have to learn to drive a wheelchair with my teeth or what?"

"Too early to tell, but your spinal cord appears to have sustained damage in the lower cervical area, so you will ultimately get some feeling back in your shoulders, arms, and hands, or you might recover much more. How much depends on you and the extent you have damaged your spinal canal."

"And just what can I do?" Although I didn't feel that I could do much of anything in my present condition.

"Be patient." Words to live by, just not *my* words.

"I'm going to get really goddamn sick of hearing that, I can tell. I think I've heard it twice today, and it's once too many."

"I can send your wife in now if you like. She's up to speed on your injuries, and she's been waiting to see you."

"Send her in," I hear myself say, unsure of what to tell her or how much she knows. The next few moments are an acid test. I feel like I'm in a situation where I can see no easy way to give it a positive spin. I have always told my wife that we were invincible as a couple. As long as we stuck together, bad things could never happen to us, but now the worst has happened. I have become a casualty, a victim, and I am the disease, not the cure. Now I understand the pity I thought I detected earlier in my wife's eyes. I hadn't imagined it. She probably knows as much as, or perhaps *more* than I do. No wonder it looked like she hadn't slept since the last time I saw her.

But this time when she enters, she smiles as if nothing is amiss. She still looks like she hasn't slept since I last saw her. I can tell because there is a strained look and redness around her blue-green eyes, but thank Christ; there is no longer any pity in them.

"Hello there," I say in my cheeriest voice as if I had just run into her on the street. It sounds horribly forced.

"Hello, Wag," she says right back in the same cheery voice. So we are two cheery little people here having a cheery little conversation; I'm wondering who will be the first to crack.

"Have you talked to the doctor?" I ask casually.

"Doctor Dumars?"

"That's his name. Did you talk to him about my condition?"

"Yep."

"That's it? 'Yep.' So, like, what did he tell you?" The forced cheerfulness is wearing thin fast. I can feel my calm unraveling.

"He told me there's a good chance you'll be just fine. But unfortunately the spinal cord swells immediately after the initial injury, which makes you temporarily paralyzed." It was just as I figured. Even if Doctor Dumars has told her everything, she has decided to hear only the positive parts.

"Did he also tell you that I broke some vertebrae?"

"Oh, sure, but that's not a big deal. The doctor says they can rebuild your vertebrae as good as new once they line up."

"But not my spinal cord." I hate that I have to make her see the downside of this situation, but I'm feeling vindictive. I've been feeling vindictive since I came out of temporary hibernation. It pisses me off that everyone else is walking, and I'm not. The worst part is that I have nobody to blame but myself, which pisses me off more than anything else—good air in, bad air out. Repeat several times. Take another inventory. Remember that this *may* not be permanent.

"Let's not think about that," she says, taking my hand and squeezing it. I know she has done this only because I can see her doing it. I find it very strange that I can see her squeezing and rubbing my hand, yet I can't feel a damn thing except a tingling in my thumb. It is somehow comforting, though, whether I feel it or not, and I'm glad she is doing it. There are so many things I want to tell her. The thoughts come all at once, but they get jammed up. There's a choke point where my brain empties into my mouth. I can't seem to concentrate on anything for very long—I suspect this has something to do with the drugs unless I have suffered some brain damage that I haven't been duly informed about. It doesn't feel like I have brain damage, but would I know if it was damaged? It is too much to consider right now. My eyes want to close, and the clouds are coming back from the ceiling. I want to drift off into the soft, smooth, spaced-out world of blissful sleep where everything will be fine, and I can forget that my head is being slowly separated from my shoulders, but there are still things I must find out.

"What happened?" I ask, not for the first time. I've pieced most of it together, but some parts of the accident are still a blur.

"I think you fell asleep. I just remember waking up, and the truck was all smashed up. I think you put your head into the sunroof. There was a ton of blood running down your neck and face. I kind of freaked out and panicked. I thought the truck would blow up, and all I could smell was gas."

"Me too," I tell her. This is one of the few things I remember: the brief remembrance of the barricade, the crash, and then the gas—the overpowering smell of gas. A scent I both like and hate. It reminds me of my dad, who would let me put gas in his truck when I was only six or seven years old. Working that gas pump felt so grown up. "I'm glad you're okay," I say, and then there's an uncomfortable pause in the conversation. I imagine both of us want to say more. But of course I have no idea what she's thinking. I'm already thinking about the restaurant and how my condition will affect the opening.

"What does the truck look like?" I don't know why I care about the truck, but it seems like the next logical question.

"Toast," she says. "It's sitting in a wrecking yard down in Lethbridge."

"Down in Lethbridge. Does that mean we aren't in Lethbridge right now?" I intuited that I was somewhere else, but I was fighting the drugs like crazy. You're not in Kansas anymore, Dorothy. It was like being high on too many 'shrooms when all you wanted was to hold onto an anchor until the storm passed and you were back in friendly waters. Everything is a new revelation. Now I know how the witch must have felt when the house landed on her. And what is with all the *Wizard of Oz* references?

"We're in Calgary, at the Calgary General Hospital," she informs me.

"Go figure," I say, trying to remember how I came to be in Calgary. The last thing I remember was being a stone's throw out of Lethbridge. We were almost home. "How did we get here?"

"By ambulance, that's how we got here," she says, trying to read my befuddled mind.

37

"Ah," I say as if everything has suddenly become crystal clear. But in reality, it is too much information. I want to go to sleep now more than ever. I have never been so exhausted; my life is too complicated. Sleeping seems like a good way to avoid thinking about it. But not before one more question.

"Who did you call?" I ask because I know my wife. When trouble surfaces, she calls people, usually someone from her rather large and supportive family. Still, considering the circumstances, she has probably called someone from my family as well, which although not as large, is just as supportive. I'm hoping she hasn't though, because I know my mother, the Queen of the Worriers, and I'm not yet ready to go to red alert. The gravity of this situation must be fully explored and mapped out before others are allowed to venture into the worry zone. I'm not ready to go to DEFCON 2 (or is it 3?). What is a DEFCON anyway?

"I called everybody," she says, confirming my worst fears. It's now ramped up to DEFCON 4. I think that's the worst one.

"Everybody, including *everybody*?" I ask, knowing my wife will understand just what I'm getting at.

"Everybody."

"How long before my mother and my family get here?"

"About three hours."

"And friends, Maple Ridgians, friends I have known for many years?"

"I phoned them about ten to twelve hours ago. I didn't know what else to do. They're driving down to see you as far as I can tell. I think Shea, Adams, and Bignell are coming."

"Shea, Adams, Bignell, and my mom all at once are a daunting prospect."

"Wag, I had to call them. I didn't know what else to do. I need someone else to talk to; this isn't easy for me."

"You did the right thing, sweetheart. I'm not mad or anything like that. I just feel too tired and sore to yap with anyone right now. So tell you what, get the nurse to shoot me full of drugs, and I'll catch a couple of hundred winks. Then I'll get my Halo shined up, and I'll be ready for visitors. By the way, what did you tell them?" I'm wondering just what she might have said because this will directly affect my mother's heart rate. She tends to overreact, which in this instance may be justified, but it is still too early to tell and much too early to release the hounds.

"I told them that you were in a serious car accident and you were in a semi-coma."

"A semi-coma. You told my mother I was in a fucking semi-coma?" My mother's heart rate would jump to about 200 beats per minute after hearing "coma" used in the same sentence as an accident.

"Well . . . you were. I didn't know what else to say." My wife tells me this, a little defensive now and more than a trifle hurt. I am an asshole.

"When they get here, tell them I'm feeling just fine, a little tired, but other than that I feel as well as can be expected considering this torture device they have attached to my head. Lie if you have to."

"Why? How do you feel—really?"

"Really? I just feel tired," I say, but to be honest, I feel like a piece of shit, like an old shoe dragged behind a car, and my future looks bleak at best, but not everyone has to know this. So memo to me: Pretend you are just fine. Deny, deny, and then deny some more. It's easier that way. I don't know it yet, but I'm going through the steps to recovery. I just got anger and denial a little screwed up. "Yep, just a little tired. Other than that, I could go ten rounds with Roberto Durán."

"Who?"

"Roberto Durán, greatest boxer who ever lived . . ." Blame it on the drugs, but I should know that my wife—although I love her dearly—wouldn't know Roberto Durán from Roberto Clemente. "Did you call *your* family?" I ask, although it is a rhetorical question.

"Yes, they send their best, and they will be here when they can but can't make it out right now."

"Understandable. It looks like I've come out of my coma anyway. Nothing to worry about here. Just keep the dogs off until I feel a little more rested." Suddenly I can no longer keep my eyes open, and I don't care enough to try. Accident, coma, what the fuck?

"Wag, you'll be okay," my wife says, sensing my distress. She stands up and plants a big kiss on my mouth, and I'm glad I can at least feel that. She looks worried, but she is putting up a good front. The woman who has been my girlfriend for nine years and is now my wife for nearly one is built of sturdier stuff than I suspected.

It is a good thing because I don't want to carry the ball right now. I'm only too happy to ride the pine and wait for the next game. "Go, team, go," I say before realizing I'm speaking aloud. I get another kiss before drifting off, thinking of my mother on an airplane somewhere over the Rocky Mountains, hyperventilating into those plastic-lined air sickness bags, trying to rationalize this setback. I think of my friends driving along the same road the plane is flying over, drinking copious amounts of frosty beverages, snacking on beef jerky, chips, and bad hamburgers at fast food joints. They will tell golf stories and discuss my current medical difficulties. They will turn a mission of mercy into a road trip. Bless all their little hearts.

CHAPTER SEVEN

BACK TO STEP ONE: DENIAL

MY ERSTWHILE COMPANION, THE I.V. pole, is looking down on me. I have decided to call him Peter—Peter Pole—it makes complete sense that inanimate objects should have names in my drugged-out and possibly brain-damaged state. First, I laugh aloud at nothing, and then the tears come. I honestly don't know what I'm crying about, and I suppose whatever drugs they're pumping into my ravaged body are working spectacularly.

My newly christened friend, Peter Pole, starts talking to me, making complete sense. After all, I have chosen to name him, thus bringing him to life. He is a mascot, but he is mine to control.

"You're awake," he says. I look around to ensure he's addressing me, but I know he's talking to me. It is the first clue I have that I am not fully awake because I cannot look around last I remember. My head does not move; it is held in place by a series of ropes, pullies, screws, and stainless steel, but the pain has decreased somewhat. Yup, give me enough drugs and I can deal with any discomfort. Bring it on. I think I could probably get out of bed and do a little dance. I took a dance class at Douglas College circa 1978, and I was damn good at it, if I say so myself. Five men and twenty-three women (girls), and what's not to like about that? But even as I relive that memory, in the back of my mind I realize I'm not going to go jiving or waltzing out of here anytime soon.

"Kinda, what's it to you?" I reply, not willing to encourage him but not entirely ready to discount him either. I'm bored and frightened; talking to an I.V. pole seems like an acceptable way to entertain myself. Better than counting ceiling tiles. In the state I'm in, I am easily entertained.

"Bit of a pansy chicken shit, aren't you?" says Peter Pole, even though secretly I know the goddamn pole isn't talking.

"Say what?" I may regret bringing him to life, but I created him, so I can also destroy him.

"You are a coward. You know what I'm talking about, C-O-W-A-R-D. Big fucking girlie-boy, take the easy way out, you cowardly coward."

"Fuck you, you skinny ass motherfucker." I am not prepared to lose an argument to an I.V pole even in my mind, although he has pretty well called it by the book. I am a coward. I'm just not about to admit it to a belligerent little undernourished I.V pole that mirrors my inner thoughts. Peter, however, will not be deterred or ignored.

"I know what you're trying to do. You're trying to sleep forever, or at least until everyone gets tired of hanging out and all your friends go home. You're avoiding the inevitable."

"So what's your point, you anorexic little stainless-steel piece of shit?" I'm not speaking per se, but Peter can read my thoughts as sure as I can read his.

"That is my point. You can't close your eyes and expect it all to go away. You can't walk. Chances are you will never walk again. Get it through your thick skull."

"A couple more hours sleep and I'll be as good as new," I insist. I truly do want to sleep forever and wake up *brand* new.

"Horseshit, and you know it. You fucked up big time, Mr. Invincible. The sooner you admit it and get on with your life, the better." I.V poles are pretty darned intuitive in this little dream world of mine.

"Fuck you," I say.

"Pardon?"

"I said fuck you and anyone who looks like you."

"Randy?"

"You heard me."

"Randy, it's me." Peter suddenly sounded an awful lot like my mother. It could mean one of two things. I was, as I suspected, not truly awake yet, or my mother was in the room. I opted for door two and brought myself back to the real world where poles can't talk or read your mind. I opened my eyes—more like I pried them open—and it was no slight relief to see my actual flesh and blood mother standing there with my wife. Two friendly, albeit worried faces.

"Mom, how are you doing? Good to see you." I still was right between planes of existence where I.V. poles talk and mothers mysteriously appear at your bedside. Drugs, especially the ones they were feeding me, pull a thin curtain over reality, and everything you do seems out of focus or done by somebody else. You know you still exist somewhere in your mind, but things move too fast and it seems like you're always playing catch up. So, it's easier just to go with the first thing that comes into your mind.

"Pull up a chair, let's talk," I say to my mother, sounding like a host on a game show. I was hoping to get out of this meeting with a minimum of histrionics. My mother is a mix of strength and perseverance, and she can be a shoulder to cry on, but she can also panic and think the worst, which brings out the big-time worrier in her. I was sixteen when I was thrown in jail for the first time one night. Assaulting a police officer was what they called it. In my mind, he deserved it, and when the police called her and told her I was in jail, she dropped like a rag doll, her bones turning to water. My older sister pointed this out later and chastised me accordingly. Police calling late at night was never a good thing. But weirdly enough, she seemed fine now, maybe because she had time to digest the seriousness of this accident. There were no tears, no blame, only motherly concern. My wife and Aunt Dorene played a supportive role in the background, and my mother seemed calm, although I could see tear tracks on their faces, which was never a good sign.

"Are you okay?" A question every good mother would ask. I went with the Demerol-induced standard answer.

"Ain't no flies on me, never felt better, chipper as a woodchuck," I lied, wondering if I was making any sense while I searched the room with my eyes as surreptitiously as possible to locate my new friend Peter Pole. I don't want him talking out of turn, but he seems to have left the party. A nurse has also appeared, and there are now four concerned faces peering down at me.

"Are you comfortable?" my mother asks, sensing my confusion.

"Truth be known, I have felt better," I belatedly admit. After all, how can you claim good health and expect to be believed while your skull is attached to numerous screws, no less, to the hospital version of the medieval rack? My neck feels three feet long. I'm hoping the nurse has appeared to give me a new shot of drugs because my tortured head begins to hurt something fierce, and the back of my neck is stretched to its breaking point. I try not to think of the pain. I try to compartmentalize the pain; compartmentalizing has always been my superpower. It's just not working so well at the moment. The immense ache is back, it's returned big-time and it's gotten worse. I mentally prescribe more drugs and more sleep for myself to zone out and leave this Kafkaesque fucking world. Wild horses are tap-dancing on my skull.

In the last two days—or three or four—I have already fallen into a pattern. I sleep three and half hours and wait in varying degrees of pain for another half-hour until the nurses come. I know it's a true half-hour because I cannot stop staring at the larger-than-life clock. They install the same clock in all schools, elementary and otherwise, so you can watch your life slip away while learning about Dick and Jane, logarithms, periodic tables, and other 'real-life' application shit. I then finally get a shot of Demerol to bring about hallucinations, confusion, and eventually blessed drugged-out sleep. I also receive a syringe of what they call Heparin or Warfarin in my gut for reasons they have not explained. It is just bizarre watching a needle go into your gut, and you can't feel any part of it. After my shots, I wait around for another four hours and start the cycle all over again. I have become institutionalized in just three short days—or four—and I am an addict.

How the cynical have fallen. Before this nasty minor accident, I had managed to "Just say no" in the last couple of years. I had sucked down or snorted most recreational drugs I could lay my hands on in my other life. But now I am a responsible future restaurant owner, so I took a dim view of drugs. But unfortunately, responsibility and recreational drugs aren't meant to mix. Good thing these drugs are totally out of my purview. They are deemed necessary, not recreational. Woohoo.

"Do you need anything?" my mother asks, reeling me back in. It is a valid question and another question any good mother would ask. I can think of a couple of flippant replies, but I swallow them. I undoubtedly need many things, but I need assurance that this is a temporary setback. I need to leap out of this hospital bed and do jumping jacks. I need to scream aloud—more than anything, I need to scream aloud—and I need to gather my strength and twist Peter Pole into scrap metal because he is an intuitive little prick. In the end, I give her the standard answer.

"Nothing I can think of. Did you have a good flight?" I listen to her pre- and post-flight adventures with forced enthusiasm. We're both on shaky ground here, juggling eggs, and God forbid any of the eggs should drop.

My mother and I are somewhat close, and we have an excellent working relationship. I tell her *some* things she doesn't like to hear, not all. She calls me an "idiot" and doesn't ask follow-up questions that would upset the status quo. I know she loves me, and the feeling is mutual, but the immediate members of our family rarely speak of inner feelings or suffer any embarrassing bouts of emotion. We all have these transient feelings, but this is not the problem. The problem is our inability to display them. Wooden hugs and firm handshakes have become our one concession in the attempt to quell all external manifestations of our heartfelt sorrows. I can tell from her expression that she would like to give me one big un-wooden hug right now, but this would produce an outpouring of sensitivity and tears that neither one of us could deal with. My defenses are way down, and so are hers.

My wife has never understood this. In her family, emotions are encouraged, even celebrated. They hug and kiss every time they meet, as if they had been apart for weeks instead of the two hours it took them to run to the store to buy a lightbulb or a pack of gum. I have learned to tolerate their ways over the years, but I am determined that it will not change me. My mother is probably more like my wife's family if push came to shove, but she is unsure how to proceed after telling me of her flight.

"I'm going to be fine," I assure her, because she needs some encouraging news, even if it is contrived. "The spinal cord swells after any contusion, and the vertebrae have to line up, and mine is no different. Doctor Dumars says I won't know anything until three months have passed." This three-month time limit seems like an excellent place to put the bar. Nobody needs to panic until two months and twenty-seven more days have elapsed. But, of course, it is an arbitrary time limit that has no meaning. I already intuit that no amount of time will heal my wounds. Still, I decide not to share my pessimistic revelations with anyone just yet, including—or is that especially—my mother, Aunt Dorene, and my understanding wife. Aunt Dorene is my mother's older sister. By all accounts, she raised my mother when my grandparents moved out of Maple Ridge, and her parents gave my mom an option to stay. She chose to stay, and her touchstone has been her sister Dorene, and somehow she has become one for me. My birthday is on Christmas Day, and my aunt always brings me something and says, "Happy birthday." A small thing that went a long way for a small kid, as she had four of her own to take care of. A slight distinction that mattered little here. I was just glad my mother's older sister was there for her.

"Fact is, I can already feel some tingling sensations in my thumbs of all places," I offered up. This part is genuine; my thumbs have begun to tingle. It's more like a general numbness between a pain and a tickle, but it is a feeling I didn't have when I last drifted off to sleep. It is somewhat annoying, like a tiny Chihuahua chewing on the end of your thumb, but it is a renewed sense of feeling nonetheless, and I'll take it any way I can get it. The woman who is my wife looks relieved but suspicious. She knows that I can be deceitful if it involves making my mother happy. She reaches out and squeezes the pad of my thumb, pinching it harder than she has to, checking for my reaction.

"Ouch," I say, on cue.

"Ouch, my ass," she says.

"No, really, I felt that. It feels like when you hit your funny bone real hard, only it's concentrated right in my thumb and kind of along the top of my forearm. It's almost like a slow-burning feeling, like when your hands are freezing, and you hold them under hot water, painful but satisfactory. That's the only way I can describe it."

"Is this a good thing?" my mother asks.

"I don't know," I say because I honestly don't. I still have a thousand questions to ask the doctor, and I don't want anyone else around when I'm asking them. But again, I will tend to err on the side of pessimism, so the disappointment I might feel when bad news is delivered won't crush me like a ball of tinfoil under the heel of a fat man's boot. I am expecting the worst and hoping for the best. I don't want a fat man squashing my little tinfoil hopes.

I catch my wife's eye for just a second while my mother is looking around the room, and I give her a look that says I've had enough and just want to be left alone. She reads the look and interprets it correctly.

"Why don't we let Wag rest for a bit, and we'll come back later. Doctor Dumars said he'd be around this afternoon, and he can answer some of the questions you might have." She sounds like a museum tour guide, but I don't care. My whole body only wants sleep right now, and if this is avoidance, then so be it. Fuck you, Peter Pole, and everyone who looks like you.

I have noticed a nurse still hovering around in the background, and if she gives me even more drugs, I will be forever in her debt. She will become my favorite person until the next time I want drugs. Such is the ebb and flow of hospital existence. Although time is relative here, and I handle Demerol well, so I'm told, and I'm not sure whether I should be proud of this or not. Unfortunately, it means I don't get morphine, although I'll take that if they want to give it to me.

My small entourage leaves the room, and my wife looks back briefly and blows me a kiss. My first instinct is to return the gesture, wave to her, and salute her somehow, but my body reminds me it is not on the same page as my brain. My hand refuses to rise even one inch off the sheet. It lies there like a dead thing.

When they are gone, the nurse approaches the bed, and I can't help but notice that she is not carrying the usual syringe full of promises and good feelings. Something has changed—she has rubber gloves on—and in one hand she is holding a couple of square blue pads the size of little welcome mats, though they look anything but welcome, and in her other hand she has what appears to be a plastic bullet. It is a fucking giant pill. I do not relish swallowing this large, cylindrical, plastic object as it looks like it could very well choke a horse, but swallow it I will if it is my lifeline to escape this reality. Unfortunately, clarity is not my cup of tea at this juncture.

But this is not the plan. This pill is not meant to be swallowed. Instead, it will be used in a way that invites just one more indignity.

A cohort has joined the original nurse, and they are speaking soothingly, much like you would talk to an alarmed, cornered animal. Just bring it on, for Christ's sake. It takes me some time to realize they are speaking to me, and while they are talking, they are gently rolling me over. They are saying something about being concerned that I have not had a bowel movement in three days, as if it is any of their business.

"This will allow you to have a scheduled bowel movement," says nurse one, holding up the lethal-looking plastic bullet generously coated with a mysterious gel-like substance.

"No, thank you," I say to her, but she is not dissuaded.

"You will receive a suppository every two days until your body becomes accustomed to a routine," she continues, "and you'll be fed stool softeners orally if necessary."

"I respectfully decline your assistance," I tell her in no uncertain terms. "I go like clockwork, if you must know, after a big-ass breakfast, one cup of coffee, and Bob's your uncle. Then I'm good for the rest of the day. Bing bang boom, so get the fuck out of my room."

"I don't think you understand, Mr. Wagner."

"Oh, I understand, alright. You and your devious assistant have conspired to stick that plastic bullet up my ass, and I, for one, am not sitting still for it." Meanwhile, sitting still was precisely what I was doing. I did not have a lot of choices in this regard. My asshole and I are essentially helpless.

"You'll need help with your bowel movements while you're here," nurse one says, "until you can do it on your own, then we'll be only too happy to stop assisting you. It won't hurt, and it will work while you're sleeping."

"I won't allow that," I say like the choice is genuinely mine. "I'll fight it. There will be no unscheduled bowel movements on my watch."

"I'm afraid you don't *have* a choice at the moment. You'll have to get used to this," and with that said, nurse one plugged the bullet into my butt. I know she did because there was a strange tingling sensation at the nape of my neck that carried up to the back of my skull, a shivery feeling that produced goosebumps up and down my arms and made my eyes open wide.

It is a sad day in my life. I cannot feel a damn thing below my shoulders save pins and needles, but they have now seen fit to violate my backside without so much as a how do you do. As a result, my most personal habits are now evidently public domain.

The catheters I have been getting since I arrived are just as intrusive. Still, their necessity was immediately apparent since my bladder was no longer draining, making me feel sick and giving me a pounder of a headache. When they first inserted a sixteen-inch hollow tube into the head of my often-appreciated dick, I was expecting severe unrelenting pain. Still, I felt nothing except that slight tingle in the back of my neck, something like the suppository. Once I drained, it immediately alleviated my headache, making the catheterizations slightly more palatable. Suppositories, though, are another thing altogether. Having strange people probe my butt, no matter how valid their arguments might be, will not be easy to forgive or forget.

Another nurse enters as they stuff the blue welcome mats underneath me, and I immediately recognize her as the drug nurse. I am saved. There are a lot of nurses, but I like her because she sticks needles into an I.V. bag, as opposed to suppositories or catheters that are much more personal. It may seem a slight distinction, but the needles don't leave me feeling violated—they are filled with happy juice. I find I require that very thing at the moment. Happy juice makes for a happy patient.

"Put me in, coach. I'm ready to play," I say and probably not for the first time. She complies and injects the Demerol in my I.V. and the Heparin into my stomach. Again, no pin-prick, no sting, nothing. It is unsettling and disturbing. The only thing *more* disturbing was the first time I watched that sixteen-inch hollow tube disappearing down the end of my dick because I could not feel it whatsoever. That whole procedure was fucking beyond unsettling.

It is not as if my dick is my life, but its importance in my life cannot be trivialized. Most times, it has served me well. But unfortunately, I have little time to contemplate these transitory thoughts as the drugs make their presence known. So, go with the good ol' happy juice, and let Captain Jack take over. Woohoo motherfucker, see you later, although who this mother-fucker might be is beyond me. I've seen fit to personify the pain.

The effect is almost Immediate. When the drug nurse has shuffled off with her needles and potions, I feel a warm, pleasant rush of blood to my head, and I am immediately floating on fluffy layers of cotton clouds. I seem to float above the bed; maybe walking is overrated anyway. It is my last thought before sleep overtakes me.

CHAPTER EIGHT

STEP TWO: MORE ANGER

WHEN I COME AWAKE AGAIN, it is dusk. I do not have an accurate concept of time. It seems like only minutes have passed since I last closed my eyes. The clock on the wall has no meaning today. It is a "transitory ticker." I remember that happening once before in day surgery some fifteen years ago when I had an operation on my bum knee. Somebody told me to count backward to ten, and voila, it seemed like not a minute had passed. You come awake slowly, and your knee is magically fixed—it occurs to me that I may have had it repaired for nothing if I can't move my goddamn legs. I wish I could stop those thoughts from coming unbidden to my mind, but they persist no matter how hard I try to drive them back. It is not negative thinking, I tell myself. It is more like reality set in.

The fog lifts slowly, and I make a concerted effort to wake up quickly because I sense someone else is in the room. I can hear people in the background. They are whispering so as not to disturb me, which makes me want to wake up even more and join the conversation. I open my mouth to let the whisperers know I'm awake, but first I must clear my throat. I manage a gruff rasping sound that erupts into a coughing fit. It is the strangest coughing fit I have ever experienced. It is more like choking than coughing. I fear I might choke to death right then and there, but I feel a sudden pressure on my stomach. It is the doctor. He pushes on my stomach again, not aggressively but decisively. My throat clears with a phlegmy hacking sound, and I barely hear the doctor's voice as I do my level best to inhale significant quantities of air. This paralytic condition in which I find myself does not allow for coughing fits or for quickly breathing in great gulps of oxygen.

"Take it easy," instructs Doctor Dumars. "You will experience some trouble coughing or sneezing for a while. Pushing on your stomach with limited force, as I have just done, will help you exhale quickly, allowing you to clear your throat. The thing is, your diaphragm is adversely affected by your spinal cord injury."

"Just how adversely is adversely?" I ask as a nurse busies herself with the blood pressure cuff.

"Well, in most cases, a breathing tube has to be inserted to clear an airway. Sometimes we use a machine for breathing if our lungs don't work independently. Your break was at the C-5, C-6 level, so a machine wasn't necessary, and fortunately you were in good shape before the accident, so breathing on your own wasn't a problem. A lot of Quadriplegics and Tetraplegics get a tracheotomy."

"Yeah, if nothing else, I sure feel fucking fortunate for small miracles," I say, causing Doctor Dumars to blush slightly. I immediately feel like an ass. My tone of voice is challenging and belligerent. He wasn't the one who steered my damned truck into a ditch, but I cannot stop lashing out at those nearby. Meanwhile, the nurse finishes taking my blood pressure, and she briefly confers with Doctor Dumars before exiting. I never hear the actual blood pressure test results, but I assume I'll live to see another day. Slow down, I tell myself, quit pissing people off. Get back to denial. It's healthier than anger.

"Your wife says you might have a few questions to ask me?" the good doctor says. He is almost shy and tentative, like he is unsure of his footing. "Oh, by the way, your bowel movement was moderately successful," he announces. I almost laugh until I realize he is serious, but I intend to avoid another coughing fit. Unfortunately, laughing leads to coughing, and coughing leads to choking. Bugger.

"I'm ecstatic," I say, the sarcasm evident because it is not a declaration I ever thought I would hear. Bowel movements are now public domain.

"What would you like to ask me?" says Doctor Dumars, evidently uncomfortable with sarcasm.

"Straight goods this time," I say. "No pulling punches, no bullshit."

"I'll try," he says.

"Okay, first off, what are the chances of me walking out of here? And none of that lip service swelling of the spinal cord fairy tale crap. Tell me upfront because I'm an upfront guy, and I don't need you to hold my hand."

"Your chances are directly affected by the damage done to the cord upon impact. The spinal cord is very delicate. For instance, if I were to drop a dime from two feet directly onto your spinal cord, it would sustain damage."

"Oh great, now I'm talking to *Bill Nye, the Science Guy*. If I could refresh your memory, I am not in here because someone dropped a dime on my spinal cord."

"Your wife said you might be difficult as time bears out your future prognosis."

"I haven't even started yet. Future prognosis, what? We're still on question one and you're hedging. So, let's make it easier. On a scale of one to ten, what are the chances of a full recovery?" He is visibly squirming now. He is the kind of doctor that prefers to deliver only good news. I believe he is too young to have seen a lot of tragedy in his life. Clean-shaven and with barely a hint of stubble, I wonder how long he has dealt with complex patients whose "prognosis" is not rosy. Hell, he had chosen to deal with spinal trauma, so he'd have to be able to talk about it eventually.

"It's hard to say," he says reluctantly. It is like dragging a confession out of a hardened secret agent trained in spy craft 101, and like a secret agent, Dumars seems only too willing to pop a cyanide tablet should the questions get more challenging. It's damn annoying.

"And my chances of a partial recovery that, best case scenario, has me walking out with a couple of crutches. I'll settle for even that."

"About half—"

"Half of what? Stick to the fucking program," I rudely interrupt.

"Four then, four out of ten, although I don't see where this is at all beneficial—"

"It's beneficial because I was never the kind of person that wanted someone to tell him his dog ran away when in reality it got run over by a fucking truck. But false hope sucks, Doc, and I don't want to be patronized for three months, or is that now two months and twenty-six days? Either way, I'll decide what to tell my wife and my mother, but I want the full story from you, which brings us back to square one. What will I fucking get back, recovery-wise?"

"That is variable," he says, visibly relieved to be back to variables. This guy would make a lousy poker player. "You will hopefully receive an operation in seven days after we make sure your vertebrae have lined up. We'll know more then, but not much more. And hope, Mr. Wagner, is all some people have. The value of hope cannot be trivialized. We hope you make a full recovery, but if you press me, I'll tell you that full recovery is unlikely after what you've gone through. I said 'unlikely,' not 'impossible,' and in my opinion, it's an exciting time to be a Quadriplegic. There is so much positive research."

"Thank you for being somewhat candid, Doc, but you can take your 'exciting time' and shove it up your ass." I have hit a nerve.

He looks nonplussed, as he should. Exciting is one stupid word to use. He takes his glasses off, blinks a few times, and tries to recover. "Doctor Dumars, if you don't mind."

"Dumars it is then," but I am so busy digesting this new information that he has already ceased to exist. He has not really told me anything I didn't suspect way down deep where real doubt slips and slinks between the rusty pilings that shore up your confidence. At least now I have a better idea of where I stand, more or less. I can't resist nailing him with one more question as he slides toward the door.

"Hey Doc, what are the chances my dick will work again? Sexually speaking, that is. Watching that tube disappear down the end of my dick without me feeling it was a scary non-sensation." His blush is almost crimson, and he isn't sure how to answer this one. His discomfort is all the answer I need. "Thanks, *Doctor Doom*," I say, lashing out once again, knowing full well this last comment will sting.

However, I don't have time to dwell on *Doctor Doom's* forecast because my mother, wife, and aunt have entered the room, and I refuse to ask dick-related questions in the presence of my mother and my aunt.

"Hi, people." I am in control once again, false bravado now quickly becoming the new normal. Never let them see you sweat. I am a rock. I am an island. "Sorry, I kind of slept away the whole day there."

"No problem," my wife volunteers while she plops herself on the corner of the bed. "We had a nice chat with the doctor, and we know you are scheduled for an operation when your vertebrae have stretched out and lined up. It seems your recovery happens, whether you are asleep or awake. Doctor Dumars seems hopeful."

"Oh yeah, he seems hopeful all right," I add sarcastically, which goes unnoticed.

The rest of the conversation is stilted and slightly uncomfortable. We try to talk as if the hospital has ceased to exist and everything couldn't be better. We steer away from any disability-related topics, as if the very act of ignoring these potential problems might make them go away. I wonder again how much information *Doctor Doom* has seen fit to share. His name will forever be in my mind as *Doctor Doom*, sworn enemy of the *Fantastic Four*. (Yes, I read *way* too many comic books in my misspent youth). All my secrets are safe with *Doctor Doom*. He has told them that an operation is imminent, so I cut the conversation short, feigning tiredness. I can almost hear Peter Pole calling me a "Yella coward" in the back of my mind as I drift off again, hoping against hope that my bones will straighten up and fly right by the time I wake up again. If I could sleep for eighty-six days in a row, then at least I would know exactly what I might be dealing with.

CHAPTER NINE

STILL STEP TWO: ANGER

TIME PASSES UNEVENTFULLY. IT DRIFTS and blends together. People come and go, and I remain blissfully stoned. Morning, afternoon, night, it's all a fucking mystery to me. All I have is that giant clock that doesn't have a.m. or p.m. But one morning (I think it's morning), there is a new development. My wife and mother wish me luck, and I am wheeled away. The next couple of hours are a blur of sustained activity. Two nurses take me down to get an X-ray, where all I see are the ceiling tiles and rows and rows of fluorescent lights with plastic casings around them. Flies have gotten into the casements because their fat, black bodies are still there, lying dead against the corrugated plastic or bashing their little fly brains out on the light cover. I know how they feel. That, coupled with the brown, rust-colored water stains on the white roof tiles, makes the hospital seem seedy and rundown. I see the hospital from a very unflattering angle. I can't help but think someone should paint catchy little messages up on the ceiling—some hope springs eternal redundancies that make you feel good about being in the hospital. Something Mallory Hopkins might say, "Life is short. Smile while you still have teeth." I arrive two floors down after about a mile of hallways, naked and barely covered by a blanket.

The X-rays are uneventful. I am drugged within an inch of insane, but I realize they have discovered that my bones have refused to cooperate.

Fuckitty fuck, they don't line up—that thought goes on forever, an earworm, "Fuckitty fuck, they don't line up"—damn vertebrae to hell and back. So I am disqualified and declared unfit for the operation. Since the X-ray was not as good as they had hoped, I can now look forward to another week in the brace that surrounds my head like scaffolding, steel wires on a Lilliputian construction site. This a grim prospect. In addition, they will add two pounds or ounces to the pulley system. I'm not sure which. I'm hoping ounces.

To make matters worse, I am informed that I am no longer welcome on this floor as I have stabilized—despite my uncooperative vertebrae—and this changes everything. It's bad enough that I no longer qualify for preferential treatment, but worse than that, I'm being turfed out of my private room and being sent upstairs pretty quick to join the general population. Being stabilized, it seems, is not such a good thing after all.

My mother, wife, and aunt are at my bedside again, so I cannot express my disappointment. Instead, I feel duty-bound to try to smile and laugh off this new development, but my smile is strained, my jaw muscles hurt like hell, and my laugh is brittle and forced. My wife notices immediately.

"It's just a different floor, Wag. But it's not the end of the world," she tells me.

"Fuck that. There are other people on this new floor. I don't like strange people," I counter in what could adequately be described as a threatening tone—as if it is partly her fault.

"Other people in the same condition as you," my mother chimed in before realizing her mistake. She has admitted that I am disabled, which is bad form, but I cannot leave my mother to twist in the wind. I do my best to appear jubilant that I am losing my private room and moving to another floor where I will be sharing a room with three other people roughly in the same condition as me, for better or worse.

"How bad can it be?" I say. "It is the seventh floor, so at least the view will improve." They laugh at this knowing full well, as I do, that the view is of no concern to me. "And the food can't get any worse," I continue, tailing off into a silence that drags on for what seems like hours.

"Wag, you're allowed to be a little depressed," my wife informs me, but I will have none of that. Depression is for wimps and whiners. So I tell myself to make a more concerted effort not to display any outward sign of distress. Never let them see you sweat. Besides, depression is like number three or four in the steps leading to recovery, and I'm not there yet.

It is something I have practiced often, making the best of a bad situation. Still, I'm informed there is only a trumped-up forty-percent chance—more or less—of walking out of here on my own power, and it is increasingly hard to appear unaffected by that forecast. Only a monumental force of will keeps me from feeling sorry for myself. Buck up, little invalid. After all, forty percent—or less—is still much better than zero, although my practical mind calls bullshit because my verts haven't lined up like little recruits in the five or six days I've been here. I wish I had a calendar in my head where I could mentally tick off days with a big black X.

"We've been up to the seventh floor," my wife says, breaking into my thoughts, "and I understand your disappointment at being moved, but . . ." and she trails off.

"But what? Tell me about it?" I ask, now mildly curious. I mean, how much different could it be? A hospital floor is a hospital floor. A room is a room, I think, with no concept of just how wrong I could be.

"Okay, so it isn't the happiest place on Earth," she finally admits. "You get off the elevator, and all these sad old people suddenly look up in expectation as if you might be their long-lost relative. Then, when they don't recognize you, their heads drop back on their chests to wait for the next elevator. It's eerie."

"They're just lonely," I say, defending these old people I have never met. I can understand why they are lonely for some inexplicable reason, and I can relate to it in a visceral way. However, I am surprised by my empathy. Usually I am not very empathetic. If anything, I tend to err way on the other side of compassion, but these old people sitting like vultures in a row have made me think of how lucky I am to be surrounded by people who make an effort to visit me. Thank goodness for small favors.

My mother, wife, and aunt stick around for another hour. They watch while a nurse feeds me. It is embarrassing, but the need for food far outstrips the demand to protect my dignity. I have already intuited that my dignity will be compromised on more occasions than I care to think about if the catheters and the morning suppository rituals I have already endured are any indications.

After feeding time at the zoo, where they spilled no small amount of strained and pre-masticated vegetables down the front of my hospital gown, my loved ones decided to leave me. They were going back to the apartment. It is only twenty minutes away, and though I say all the necessary things to make them feel as though I can carry on without them, they hesitate, like they are deserting me. But eventually they relent, and I am glad to see them go. I need time to contemplate my future without legs that work, without a dick that works, and drugs that make I.V. poles come alive. On top of that, now I have a room with a view and roommates I didn't ask for, but I will just consider it another adaptation in a long line of adaptations. One more small wrinkle to iron out in my already wrinkled-up environment. The theme is evident here. It seems the only way to survive is to roll with the punches. It's rope-a-dope time, folks, and I am just hoping against hope that the opponent wears himself out before I go down for the count. The punches come fast and furious in this place. It would be too easy to let my guard down and give myself over to the canvas, but things are bound to improve. Clutch and grab. Get your breath back. My life has become a colossal boxing metaphor, and I am fighting it out with my fucked up spinal cord.

It is not yet time to panic. There will be plenty of time for that later. I'm informed that my move has been delayed, but I don't ask why. Instead, I ask for more drugs, and I am told the next shot is several hours away. This delay does not sit well, and I react before I can help myself. "Fuck you then, who needs fucking drugs anyway," I say, knowing it is a childish remark. I still feel better after I have said it, even though they are the procurers and the administrators of the drugs keeping me alive, or leastwise semi-happy to be alive. I bite back the rest of my comments and try to be patient, but some pain just can't be trivialized. Yes, they have reattached the goddamn pulley. A pulley with extra weights.

Despite the pain, my mind wanders, and I find myself close to sleep, drifting in and out in a dreamlike state, only somewhat aware of my surroundings. It is an excellent way to whittle away the hours until my next drug fix. I am floating again. Once more, I am above the bed, looking down at the pitiful creature I have become, and while I watch, I can see my body shrinking. It is slowly withering away. The physique I spent the last thirty years agonizing over folds in on itself as muscle mass melts off my bones. My chest caves in, and my hands curl into claws. I stare in disbelief at what my body is becoming, and if I could scream out loud, I would. Even without control of my diaphragm, I give it a shot anyway, but the sound is not overly loud, and I fail to attract anyone's attention.

All I have succeeded in doing is bringing back the pain tenfold. I try to localize it to one spot and send it to the part of my brain that lies behind closed doors. I am quickly learning pain management: mind over matter. I am succeeding somewhat when I become aware of another presence in the room.

At first, I suspect it is another visitation from Peter Pole, but when the presence asserts itself, I can see it is indeed a man standing next to my bed. A man dressed entirely in black, save for a small inauspicious white-collar surrounding his throat. He looks an awful lot like an undertaker, and I take great pains to remind him in no uncertain terms that I am still very much alive and perhaps he could come back tomorrow.

"No, no," he says, smiling with big capped white teeth borrowed straight out of a Pepsodent commercial. "It is not like that at all. I was just hoping we might have an informal chat. Nurse Chalmers thought that perhaps I might give you a spiritual lift. She tells me you have a lot of questions, and I might be able to offer you some comfort. So if there is anything you wish to discuss, please feel free to bring it up, and rest assured that whatever you might say will stay in this room. Confidentiality is assured."

"And just who the fuck are you? And give Julia Roberts her teeth back. You're freaking me out." I consider this a reasonable suggestion.

"I'm a Catholic priest. Father Delwinny. We have a small church down on the bottom floor. When you're well enough, you might see fit to visit us."

"Not fucking likely. I'm not a big believer, and that's putting it lightly. In truth, I am anything but a *big* believer. I am a one hundred percent died-in-the-wool atheist heretic," I tell him. I have gone out of my way to rail against the gatekeepers of so-called organized religion. They are charlatans, altar boy diddlers, and money grabbers that fleece and cajole disenfranchised people of their hard-earned cash. They use God as a tool and eternal damnation as a threat. I despise them and their arrogance. In short, I don't like 'em much.

"Things change," he says. "We all come to God in the end."

"Yeah, when pigs fucking fly, pal."

"Pardon me. I'm sorry if I offended you." He is taken aback by my vehement reaction. I had put a wrench into what was likely building up to a rah-rah, sis-boom-bah God speech.

"You're sorry," I say, taken aback by his sad sense of surprise as if everyone should consider God's presence eventually, and then the rant starts all over again. I have found a patsy for my anger.

"No, you should be sorry. What kind of stinking God would let me fall asleep while driving, allowing me to break my neck in the prime of my life? Bother somebody else. Oh, and if you see a nurse, send her in. They're my first line of defense, and they're doing a pretty shithouse job letting you in here." He starts to get up, but he still looks uncertain. His hands flutter about his face. They are like small birds with no place to land, no perch to rest. I have run out of energy, but somehow I feel better, even though it has come at the expense of a person that only wishes to spiritually comfort me. I'm now totally spent. His hands can now roost as he leaves, walking backward and bowing at the waist. I know I have not endeared myself to him or his God, but he has picked the wrong time to approach me—once I stop breathing would be the only good time. I may not believe in God, but I sure have no trouble blaming him for my current predicament.

Five or six short days ago, I would have relished the idea of going toe to toe with one of God's little mindless disciples, but now I tire easily, and I have no more venting to do. I just needed a direction for my hate, and the priest has come in handy. The amount of hate that builds up underneath the façade of normalcy is incredible. I cannot construct a dam big enough to hold it all in.

The head nurse replaces God's errand boy. At least I think she's the head nurse. She has taken the reins, so to speak, and I consider her to be my primary caregiver. Hence, she is also directly responsible for any discomfort I might feel.

"Hey Florence," I forget her real name, and the tag's obscured, "try to keep the riff-raff out, will you? Or do you get a bird dog fee for successful converts?"

"Funny guy," she says in a tone that leads me to believe she doesn't find me even remotely funny. "That poor guy was just trying to help you out. He does some good work in the hospital."

"Look, if I'm destined to end up in his version of hell, I'll have plenty of time to regret my words and actions later. So I don't need your help."

"Some people find the notion of a benevolent God comforting."

"Well, some people are fucked in the head. Even a brain injury wouldn't screw me up that badly. Religion is the opiate of the huddled masses, I read that or something like that somewhere, and it wasn't in the Bible."

"Your wife told me you don't usually swear as a rule, and it lists Roman Catholic as your religion of choice on your admitting form. I just thought you might benefit from a little spiritual diversion. I won't make that mistake again."

"My wife is telling the truth in one respect; I don't usually swear, but it just seems so damned appropriate in this place. I think swearing is helping to preserve what's left of my sanity. And I'm not Catholic, Roman, or otherwise, even though my wife no doubt indicated I was. I lied on my marriage certificate so I could be married in a Roman Catholic Church. Hah, I even said I would bring my kids up to be good little Roman Catholics. What a crock of shit."

"You're allowed to be afraid."

"I'm not afraid," I say, thinking that she has just hit the proverbial nail on the head. I am afraid. I'm worried I won't get any better and someone will be taking care of me for the rest of my life. I'm afraid because I'm too young to be disabled. I'm afraid, anxious, angry, depressed, and scared in spades, but this should not be apparent to the nurse. It must remain my secret because emotions must be held in check at all costs. That first rock that tumbles down the side of the mountain could start a landslide, which could conceivably bury me.

"You're going through one of the first steps," says the nurse, smiling now, enjoying my consternation. She has taken on another tone now, the tone of someone wise and world-weary. Fuck steps. Although I realize they have documented this grieving process, everyone is different. Nevertheless, I decided to listen to her version.

She is probably years younger than I am and pretty in a homespun way. No makeup, some freckles, an innocent smile, and dimples that make her look cute instead of classically beautiful. Her strawberry-blond hair, tied back with a red cloth elastic, hasn't been teased or manufactured. At the same time, as I'm trying to judge her age, I'm also trying to see through her uniform because she has a great body. Just because your dick is dormant, your appreciation for the female form doesn't disappear. She has already told me that she has been down this path before and that I am not the first patient she has had with a damaged spinal cord. I finally read her nametag. Nurse Chalmers has more going for her than just a snazzy uniform and a reasonable bedside manner. Even though she is the same nurse who sicced the priest on me, I find her very understanding and likable. Her tone and demeanor are calming.

"First steps of what?" I ask. "Sorry about that, but start again. I kind of zoned out on you." I'm interested but, as always, skeptical.

"Of recovery. The steps of recovery."

"Oh yes, the specific steps of recovery," I say, trying not to sound snide and doubtful.

She continues unabated. I don't think she can be rattled easily, and she starts again. "So, I've been led to believe, and in most cases, it seems to run true to form that there are five steps of recovery. First, there's denial—"

"Well, that isn't me," I interrupt with barely disguised cynicism. "In no way can I deny that I am lying in a hospital bed fucked over for good and may never walk again, let alone wipe my ass or brush my teeth."

"So you say. The second step is anger, then bargaining—"

"Bargaining? What kind of step is that? Is that like where you promise you'll lead a monk's life, never spit on the sidewalk, covet thy neighbor's wife, jerk off, or stick gum under a chair ever again if only you could walk?"

"Something like that, but in a more spiritual sense. It's more like repenting to get what you want. Like promising ridiculous things in return for recovery. Making bargains with God or a higher power."

"Back full circle to this religious horseshit again." I can't help but roll my eyes, but even that gives me a head rush. They're feeding me the good drugs.

"It means different things to different people." She shrugs her shoulders then and straightens my pillow and blankets while I try to look down her blouse—maybe my dick is not as dead as I first thought, or perhaps it's just what guys do. I'm going with the latter. She leaves me to think about these two steps I have supposedly been going through. I make a note to quiz her about the final two steps, but for now my mind is preoccupied with these first three revelations.

"Denial," I say. The word is said out loud more than once. I'm getting the feel of it, as if saying it repeatedly will give me some new understanding of the concept of it. I don't think I'm in denial, but maybe this is all part of being in denial in the first place; not admitting the denial. So in essence, I deny my denial. This is an awful *Catch-22*. I make another mental note to keep deep thoughts to a minimum while on Demerol.

My addled brain is finally tired, but it gets to work on the next two steps. First, anger, a natural reaction. But bargaining? I decide to say that word out loud. I am like a parrot that has just learned how to talk. "Bargaining," I say slowly, and while that word rolls off my tongue, I am thinking just what I would personally sacrifice to be up and walking again. First, would I give up drinking? I decide that's a no-brainer since drinking probably contributed to my downfall in the first place. Second, would I give half my money to charity? I chuckle to myself over this since half of zero is still zero. Would I kill someone? Ooh, now there's the big brain bender. Now we're getting somewhere.

"Would I kill someone?" I'm speaking out loud again. It is an annoying habit, and I'm hoping it is a habit that will eventually pass on its own. I write it off as a symptom of the brain damage I may have sustained. However, it makes me think of the stitches they told me about that reside in the back of my head due to my abrupt attempted departure from the truck's cab, which makes my head itch where I imagine my stitches would be. It is an itch that I have no hope of scratching, and thinking about it hurts my Halo.

I decide to forego whether I would kill someone for now because it will require more thought than I am willing to give, and my head hurts like a motherfucker. I have decided it is drug time, happy hour has arrived, and my brain can now take an official time out.

But just as I finish this thought, I hear a commotion out in the hallway. If I'm not mistaken, my friends from Maple Ridge have arrived. Better late than never.

CHAPTER TEN

DENIAL AGAIN,
I CAN'T SHAKE IT

A NURSE IN THE HALLWAY briefly holds them up, but they are a force of nature and they come blowing into my room on a wave of boozy hellos, loud exclamations, and good intentions. Shea leads the delegation.

"Wagner. How the fuck are you?" he says until he sees the Nautilus machine attached to my head like an alien insect, and the abrupt realization that I am not doing well at all hits him like a lead pipe upside the head. His expression changes mid-sentence, and I know he is not fully prepared to see me lying helpless in traction in a hospital bed. I wonder how much my well-meaning wife has told him.

He seems perplexed and nonplussed. It takes everything he has not to turn around and bolt, but with a concerted effort he pulls himself together and sidles up to the bed. Shea is a strange mixture of gruff nonchalance and bravado, which effectively belies his capacity for deep abiding concern. He has a poignant wit and can be loyal to the point of distraction. All his hard edges become rounder and softer the longer you know him. He is like a small bear. I have known him for a long time.

I met Shea about twenty-plus years ago when I was actively pursuing the affections of one of his sisters. He has three beautiful sisters, and I deemed each one worthy of my respect (although these affections were not always reciprocal), mainly because I was a young guy whose hormones were doing all the thinking for him. Shea's sisters were not hard to look at, to say the least, and they sure as hell deserved better than me.

Shea was always around when I'd drop by his mother's place to expend misguided energy on his sisters, and we grew to be friends. Now, some two decades later, I can't tell you whatever became of his sisters, and I don't spend much time worrying about them, but I came away with a good friend in Dan Shea, who has stuck with me over the years and will likely be around when and if we live long enough to become old. I have probably lived with Shea and shared an apartment or basement suite with him longer than any other friend. We always ended up in the same place, from Calgary to Maple Ridge. If you hang around with Shea, you'll never be bored.

However, Shea is still tongue-tied, and I should say something to relieve the apparent tension, but I can't seem to think of anything befitting the situation. Witty banter and Demerol share a different space and time. Besides that, I have no precedence to draw from. I am an empty well, and I look rather helpless and pathetic. There is not much I can do or say that will immediately allay his obvious misgivings. These are my close friends, and I can't easily lie to them without them knowing it, so I don't even try.

"I feel like I look," I manage to say before Shea steps aside, and the room is filled with Adams and Bignell, who both look mildly overwhelmed but not out of their depths. Of course, they have received a more thorough briefing than Shea, or they mask their emotions better. But on the other hand, I have known them a lot longer, and they wouldn't hesitate to express their concerns openly should they have any.

"Boy, you look like someone who came out on the losing end of a fight that involved instruments of torture and large blunt objects," says Bignell, managing to state the obvious in a skewed way that is so much a part of his personality.

"Thanks, my little friend, and trust you to put the way I feel into words." Some would say Bignell is eccentric, bordering on strange, but it is a trait I have come to accept in him. We probably get along as well as we do because I forgive him for his quirkiness as he forgives me of my many idiosyncrasies.

He is another old friend that goes back over twenty-plus years. We were near inseparable through high school, inseparable but diverse. He was prone to excesses, and while his tormented soul kept him forever on edge, I was forever mellow, a referee, and, in retrospect, probably quirky in my own right but grounded in comparison. He was angst incarnate, where I was convinced of my superiority, perhaps because I genuinely lacked *inner* confidence, but I projected the opposite. Bignell was also obsessive to the point of being institutional, where I tended (and still do) to go with the flow. It required an inordinate amount of energy to be Bignell's closest friend. My role in our relationship was to play mediator and frequently savior as little stood between him and inevitable chaos.

In what I refer to as "the early disturbing years," people around him were either burned up or burned out very quickly. But despite all our differences, or because of them—for reasons neither one of us felt compelled to explore or explain—we complimented each other quite well, although our relationship could be classed as clearly antagonistic.

I first met him at a mutual friend's house. Ray Herman and I started the day playing an uninspired one-on-one basketball game until Bignell showed up. It then deteriorated quickly into a huge wrestling match between Bignell and myself, where the only real casualty was his nerd-boy white cardigan sweater. However, Ray Herman had the good sense to stand down and watch.

The wrestling match started because of Bignell's steadfast refusal to play by any organized basketball rules. So instead, we engaged in something akin to rugby and wrestling, with a pinch of basketball thrown in, where there was no such thing as rules. As far he was concerned, the usual traveling violations, double dribbles, or personal fouls had no place on a backyard basketball court. Thankfully the court was grass, or neither of us would have any skin left.

What we engaged in couldn't really be called basketball, save that there was a hoop involved. Instead, it was more a game of attrition with muddled, adaptive rules where the sole object of the game was only to put the ball into the hoop at any cost. I remember that I did manage to come out slightly ahead in the contest, but only because I had a rudimentary knowledge of the derivative game, more natural ability, and a slight height advantage. Bignell was built like a gymnast. He was of proportionate muscle, five-foot-four at twelve years old, great for balance but not great for leaping. He did not accept my marginal victory graciously. Instead, it made him determined to prove his prowess with games I was not so familiar with. So, after much haranguing and verbal jousting, we scheduled a sports day of sorts the very next week to be held at his place, where we would play lesser-known games such as ping-pong, weightlifting (only Bignell could turn that into a game), eight-ball, darts, and karate.

Bignell may not have been inclined to play organized sports like most other children, but his proficiency at sports that required self-motivation soon became evident.

I was thrashed on the pool table and soundly whooped at darts; although I did manage to represent my neighborhood well in ping-pong and in the weightlifting competition, I still fell woefully short. But where I truly took a good kicking, both literally and figuratively, was in an impromptu karate match. I was punted in the head twice with roundhouse kicks that jarred my teeth and jaw right down to my Stan Smiths.

It was the beginning of a beautiful friendship. From then on, we each played to our strengths. I tended to apply myself to organized team sports, and Bignell continued to kick my ass in pool and darts. After that, we split pretty evenly on karate until he took it upon himself to achieve certified belt dominance. Fortunately, by then we had passed that stage in our relationship where we felt inclined to roundhouse and snap-punch the living bejesus out of each other.

While I was contemplating and my mind wandered off, Bignell, Adams, and Shea had exchanged surreptitious glances. I feel I am on the sideline somehow, even though it is not hard to figure out that I am the sole object of their evident anxiety.

"So, where should I start?" I finally ask to break up the pregnant pause. I fucking hate pregnant pauses and tend to fill them with any inanity that pops into my brain, but nothing about this seems inane.

"Wherever you're comfortable starting," says Adams, forever polite. He is the oldest of all my friends. Not in age but in the time we have spent together. I cannot remember a time when he hasn't been there.

We grew up on the same street, right next door to each other, separated by a short picket fence. Adams's mother and my mother were both starting families at about the same time, and it was often hard to tell whose kids were whose as we grew up. I had spent most of my waking moments with Adams as we went from diapers into grade school. From there, when many people tend to go their separate ways, we remained joined at the hip, and we are still united in a way that only people who have spent a lifetime together can understand. He is no less my brother than my actual flesh and blood brother. He reached his full height of about six feet plus early in life. He started shaving when he was about twelve, whereas I believe I started shaving at about twenty. Adams could grow a beard in three days, and he insisted on sideburns, giving him that "Elvis" look and making it very easy for him to bootleg for the crew. At seventeen, we took a road trip to California, and he was going into liquor stores even down there, where the age to purchase was twenty-one. I don't remember him ever having to produce I.D. after his sixteenth birthday.

Adams will always be the voice of reason. When I zigged, he contemplated. When I zagged, Adams procrastinated. We invariably arrived at the same destination, but he would expend less energy and frustration to get there. While I experimented, Adams accumulated data. Although eight months younger, he would always be the more mature and measured one. I had little or no boundaries. Where I would drop the gloves and start swinging, he would consider, plan, and swing only as a last resort. Adams invariably preferred discussion to action without provocation.

Adams was not unlike that old animated standby, *Fred Flintstone*, when the time came to dream up a get-rich-quick scheme. And once he set his mind on something, he was one of those highly motivated guys that kept his focus. Were we not pushed together as children, it is doubtful we might have ever met at all, but meet we did due to a geographical fluke that put our mothers on the same street. Our friendship has endured, withstanding the test of time.

"What are you looking at?" I finally say to Adams, who has continued to stare at me since he came into the room.

"Just digesting," he says like he's playing chess, and the next move might decide the very outcome of the match.

"Not much to digest here," I say. "What you see is what you get. I screwed up on a large scale, and now I'm playing the time-will-tell game."

"Can you feel this," says Bignell, semi-softly jamming a finger into my ribs.

"Nope, can't feel fuck all from about the collarbones on down, give or take a tingle here and there. That ought to postpone our next sports day indefinitely."

"How indefinitely?" says Bignell, sounding concerned, undoubtedly sadly envisioning a day in the future where he can no longer exercise his right to roundhouse kick me to the head.

"*Doctor Doom*, the resident perpetually optimistic physician, has given me a three-month time limit, at which point he will deem me fit or unfit for complete recovery depending on what sensation returns." I decide not to share my misgivings with them at this time. If I know Adams, he will quiz the doctor relentlessly at the first opportunity anyway and find a quiet corner to read up on the subject. Bignell will not believe the doctor. Instead, he will wait for a quiet moment when we are alone, and he might address the problem up-front with a series of questions that will leave little doubt about how I think and feel about the whole thing. Shea will absorb information through osmosis until all is said and done and will then come to his own conclusions, valid or otherwise, and will be the first to put it into perspective. Shea always had a skewed view, but he was rarely wrong. He would be the first one to cry when no one was looking.

My wife comes in now, and I think this must be hard for her, not for the first time. Then, finally, all conversation ends while she hugs each guy in turn. She looks visibly relieved. My mother has been in town for a while, and today she decided to stay at our apartment in Calgary and would see me tomorrow. They have planned a barbecue back at headquarters, assuming safety in numbers. So what my mother has essentially done is taken a moment to regroup, and I'm secretly sure that Shea, Adams, and Bignell will do the same once they are all hanging out.

We talked for a couple of hours about mundane things: the weather, the things that have changed in Maple Ridge since I last checked in, the progress of our new restaurant, and why Walker (another friend who goes back many years) couldn't make it. No time off work. Walker is one job-responsible guy. We jabber about neutral things because nobody wants to upset the bedridden guy. There will be plenty of time to discuss the bedridden guy when the bedridden guy isn't around. Bignell is the only one who is clearly uncomfortable with this unspoken concession. He is squirming with unanswered questions.

The bedridden guy is not concerned; however, he only wants another hit of drugs and some serious nap time after a couple hours of conversation. I finally bid them farewell and told them to relax at the apartment and not worry about coming back that night, as I would see them tomorrow. Every day I get a little stronger, I assure them, and they all shuffle out, except my wife, who stays behind to kiss me and tell me that she loves me. She is near tears now and will probably let the dam burst on the drive back to our tiny apartment. However, she has shoulders to lean on now, and she is immensely relieved. Consequently, I am relieved for her.

Nurse Chalmers—what the hell is her first name?—is hovering this time because she has a schedule to keep. I am probably not the only cranky drug addict she has to deal with.

I take one in the gut to thin my blood and one in the drip for pain. It takes mere minutes until I can feel the comforting, blissful fog closing in, and my body starts to shut down. My brain is only minutes away from the fluff cycle. I'm in the process of deciding what I'll dream about—one of the anomalies of Demerol is that you can almost handpick your dreams—when I feel a hand on my shoulder gently shaking me back into the land of the aware.

It seems Ron Bignell has returned, or maybe he never left, but he is here with me in my drugged-out state.

CHAPTER ELEVEN

STEP THREE, BARGAINING

I'M NOT HAPPY ABOUT BEING semi-awake. It's a buzzkill for sure. "Go away. I have bigger fry to fish," I say, obviously confused, but Bignell is persistent. It is in his D.N.A.

"Yeah, right, like I drove out here to have a barbecue; not bloody likely. I can barbecue in my own backyard, thanks."

"Where you can make up all your own rules, you and your fucking cardigan," I finish for him, clearly losing ground to the effects of Demerol.

"I drove out to see how you're handling this shit, and don't give me any of that 'I am a rock, I am an island' crap you usually spew. Instead, I want to know why your hands, arms, and basically the rest of your body don't work and what the hell happened."

"I crashed," I say, hoping this will be a sufficient explanation. I should be so lucky.

"I know you crashed. I know you fell asleep. I even know they put all that hardware on your head to straighten out your spine so you can get ready for an operation. What I don't know is how you feel about the whole thing. You know your body better than anyone. So, how come it isn't working up to fresh-from-the-factory standards anymore?"

I close my eyes briefly, real tight, and open them again to make sure he is really there. I would almost prefer to talk to Peter Pole right now. But when he doesn't disappear, I decide there is little choice but to speak with him until either he goes away or I do. Besides, I tell myself, it might feel good to talk out loud about some of my fears and doubts. So I decided to vent a little, or a lot, depending on where the mood took me. Bignell won't press very hard once I start. He will let me vent only as much as I need or want to.

"The thirty-year warranty on this body has expired, and I truly think I'm fucked up for life," I start, giving him an idea of possible scenarios. "I've separated my vertebrae and damaged my spinal cord, which is not a good thing, and after conferring with *Doctor Doom*, you know the guy from—"

"Yeah, yeah, the *Fantastic Four* villain. Remember, I read the same comic books. Go on," he says to hurry me up. He is quite possibly the only person who has read as many comics as me, but talking fast is not in my bailiwick. Demerol will not allow it.

"Well, like I was saying, I've been led to believe that spinal cords don't repair themselves. They don't want to fucking heal, is what I'm saying. They don't mend. They stay fucked up even after the bones around them get a remake, and after three months, I might be able to feed myself and scratch my head, which incidentally itches like fucking crazy." I move my scalp around by wiggling my ears, hoping to alleviate the itch slightly. My hair has not been washed for seven days (my best guess). My eyebrows arch up and down, making my ears wiggle, but the itch persists. All I've done is aggravate my neck. It's suddenly all I can concentrate on. It no longer matters that I may never get another woody or take an unscheduled crap. All that matters is that someone scratches the top of my head. Bignell reads my distress, and he massages my head between the monkey bars and the screws. It doesn't strike me as weird that he gently scratches my head. If I could do it myself, then what he is doing might be construed as abnormal.

"Man, that feels great," I say. "What sucks the big one is that I can't do any of this shit myself. Scratch my head, feed myself, brush my teeth, or even floss. Hell, I can't even pick my nose." My thoughts are leaking out again and forming themselves into words and escaping without me giving them the green light to do so.

"So just ask. What's the big deal? Except I might have to draw the line on that pick-your-nose thing."

"Oh yeah, easy for you to say. It's all fucked up in my book. I've made it a point to never ask for anything in my life, and now suddenly I have to ask for everything. I have to be fed, for Christ's sake. They brush my fucking teeth with giant flavored Q-tips, wipe my ass, and even drain my bladder. It's like being a goddamned newborn baby with a working brain and a body I have no control over. It sucks big, hairy dick."

"So, then it gets easier, and maybe before you know it you can brush your own teeth and wipe your own ass, but for now you've got to go with it because you don't have a choice." By that time, he had stopped scratching my head and had moved back around where I could see him. He gives me his best "what are you going to do?" big-ass shrug and a helpless out-of-his depth look. He has thought about how much movement I'm going to get back.

"I just hadn't figured this into the rest of my life," I tell him. "I always had this attitude, you know, like I was destined for greatness or something, like this kind of shit only happened to other people. In my mind, that meant I was immune to this kind of setback." The drugs were kicking in big-time now, and my thoughts were coming hard and fast, but blurry. All glimpses into the future hinged on the possibility that I would not improve. I focused on that, which prompted me to ask an unexpected, perfectly reasonable question.

"Would you kill me if I asked you to?"

"Would I kill you?" He looked at me like I'd lost my mind, and it's hard to surprise Bignell.

"Yeah, you know, pull the plug. Kevorkian me. End my puny little existence?"

"Right now, you mean?" and he looked around like he was getting ready to do that very thing.

"No, Jesus Christ. Not right now. I'm not in that big of a hurry. It's just that I don't know if this is all I'll get back, so you'd be killing me a little prematurely at this point. I'm talking about later, after all the chickens come home to roost and every option has been explored." I must have looked serious, or he wondered what role chickens might play in this scenario. He gave it solemn consideration before he answered.

"Probably not," he finally says.

"Probably not . . . maybe? Or probably not for sure?"

"Probably I'd have to really fucking think that one over. It depends, I guess. For instance, if you could somehow defend yourself, then I might be able to kill you. But certainly not if you're defenseless. I couldn't kill you if you couldn't fight back."

"That makes zero fucking sense. Think about it. If I could defend myself, I could no doubt kill myself." We are quiet until another thought occurs to me, and I blurt it out. "Just a minute, Adams is supposed to kill me. Problem solved."

"What?" He isn't making the same jumps as I am. He isn't keeping pace. I have to stop and remind myself that the rest of the world isn't being shot full of Demerol at four-hour intervals.

I continue, and I'm pretty happy with myself for solving this problem. "When we were young, like ten or something, Adams and I talked about this very thing. We decided that should either one of us end up a vegetable, the other one would be duty-bound to end his life. He would have to kill me. He promised, and I couldn't very well take his job away without asking him. Forget I asked *you* because, as it turns out, I did ask him first. So it seems only right to give him the first right of refusal."

"You were kids. It's not the same," he says, sounding almost like he's about to make a case for himself as the right guy for the job. Like he's just failed an interview, and he has to salvage something out of the exchange. "And besides, you're not a vegetable . . . not yet, anyway."

"Uh-huh, right. So, what can I do that, say, an acorn squash or a pumpkin couldn't do?"

"An acorn squash or a pumpkin? Where the hell did you come up with that? That's not a valid comparison," he says, clearly not entirely satisfied with my vegetable selection, like I had an entire supermarket of vegetables to choose from, and I chose wrong. There's just no pleasing some people, but he looks dumbfounded. He scratches his head before saying anything else, an innocent gesture that makes my head itch again.

"Well, for one thing, you can reason. Acorn squash or pumpkins can't reason."

"Do I sound reasonable?" I ask, wondering, and not for the first time, if I would know if I were brain damaged. Indeed, someone would have picked up on that by now.

"No, not particularly reasonable. Do you know something I don't?"

"Well, the way I see it, I've got about as much to live for as an acorn squash." For some reason, this makes him laugh. It isn't the response I was looking for, as I thought I'd just made a very valid point.

"What kind of drugs are they feeding you?"

"Demerol. But not enough, not nearly enough."

"Before we continue this conversation, maybe I ought to get a shot of that shit, so we're on the same page." Then he brings his hand to his chin again and scratches his three-day-old beard in thought. It makes my chin itch in turn. Adams and he both have this annoying habit of rubbing their chins while pondering their next move. It should be a new rule, no scratching or rubbing of any kind around the vegetable boy.

"You aren't about to ask Adams to kill you either," he finally says, making me wonder doubly hard what the hell we were talking about since Demerol makes my brain mushy. While he was scratching his chin, I had gone on a drug-fuelled excursion somewhere. I almost forget Bignell is there. "Besides that, he never would. You know that as well as I do." I open my mouth to speak, but he is no longer paying much attention to me, and my mouth shuts before the words come out. I allow him to continue unchallenged. "Now, I don't doubt that you could probably kill Adams should the situation be reversed, so maybe it's a good thing it's you laying there instead of him, but asking *me* to kill you after six days does seem a little harsh."

"I didn't ask you to kill me. I asked if you were capable of killing me. There's a fuck of a lot of difference there. I want to be sure we're clear on this point before I go to sleep."

"So you're thinking ahead, in a manner of speaking."

"Well, yeah, I'm thinking ahead. Hence the acorn squash and pumpkin reference."

"Enough with the goddamn vegetables already. Let's stick to what we know, which isn't a heck of a lot. The way I see it, what you have to do here is—"

"If you say 'be patient,' I'll scream for the guards. I've had 'be patient' up to here," and I begin to laugh because I can't make the cutting motion with my hand at neck level to let him know where exactly I've had it up to. My wrist flexes, but I can't lift my arm, let alone my whole hand, and somehow it hurts my head to try.

"Be patient is good advice. I don't know what else to tell you. I do realize it's something you don't exactly excel at."

"I don't have patience. Is that what you're saying? Well, I call bullshit. I've got more than you fucking know, but I must admit, it feels like I've been lying here for four years instead of five days—or is it six? No matter, five or six, it makes little difference. The point is, I'm still polite to people. You try being patient while someone is greasing up a rubber glove in preparation to invade your body cavities."

"No thanks, I'll pass. But it sounds interesting . . . Did you tell your wife any of this shit? About you thinking you're not going to get any better? About Adams promising to kill you should you fail to improve?"

I'd had enough of visiting. "Nah, that shit just came up for the first time. You bring out the best of me. Now, haven't you got somewhere to be that isn't even close to here right now? Because I don't want to think about the future anymore. I'm through venting, and I'm double-dog friggin' tired."

"You can't shut her out, you know."

"Fuck that for now. I'm willing to pretend I'm getting better when my wife, aunt, and especially my mother are around."

"And later on?"

"Later, Adams might agree to kill me. That is if you don't talk me to fucking death. In the meantime, I am now triple dog-tired, one ahead of double-dog. So go away and let me get back to feeling sorry for myself. It requires my full concentration. You have no idea."

"Okay, if you're determined to go to sleep, go ahead. I'll just sit here for a while if you don't mind."

"Me laying here being paralyzed is screwing with your brain, isn't it?"

"Yeah, it is."

"Yeah, mine too, scares the shit out of me."

"Well, whatever it takes. You know people are pulling for you and all that shit, and I speak for a lot of people."

"Fuck you. You never spoke for anyone else in your life. That's just hospital talk about making me feel better—bedside banter. I'm sick to death of that shit. Go keep 'em busy while I sleep."

"Okay, so I speak for just me. Anything you need, just ask, except for killing you. I'm not ready to do that just yet."

"Go away."

"Okay." And I waited with my eyes closed, listening for his footsteps, but I could still feel him beside me.

"Are you still here?" My eyes had been closed for what felt like hours.

"Go to sleep."

"I can't. You're looking at me."

"How do you know? Your eyes are closed."

"With Demerol, you can see through your eyelids."

"Okay, how many fingers am I holding up?"

"More than me."

"Good answer."

And then I must have reached out and again caught the Demerol express to dreamland because it's the last thing I remember.

CHAPTER TWELVE

STEPS TWO AND THREE:
ANGER AND BARGAINING

I SLEEP WELL FOR CLOSE to three hours. I know it's only been three hours because that's all the sleep the nurses allow me. They are duty-bound to turn me and put pillows under my back, and it only hurts when you breathe. There are many "duties" when taking care of a Quad. Flipping and rolling me like a well-trained Judo team is necessary so I don't get any bedsores, but fuck me if I don't feel the screws in my head scraping the bones in my skull where the Halo is attached every time they do it.

They are always polite about it. The nurses ask me whether I want anything to drink. If I answer yes, they fill me up with water, or cranberry juice if they can find it; cranberry juice is the best thing to drink in the ongoing struggle to avoid bladder infections, so I am told. Unfortunately, if I drink, this means that on the next turn, instead of just rolling me over like a big old log, they stick a drainage catheter into the end of my dick and chart my liquid output and analyze my urine like little mad scientists. Now I'm barely awake when this happens, and it serves as just another small reminder that I'm becoming institutionalized.

The night passes quickly in three-hour intervals, and the following day while enjoying that blissful one-hour of false dawn before the inmates start stirring, I try again to move parts of my body, and this time I meet with a bit of success. As near as I can tell, my wrist can now bend backward a little more, and I can move my fisted hands up and down. I just can't seem to lift the palm-up side of my hand. It rolls, but it doesn't raise. After much experimentation, I learn to bug-walk my hand almost up to my chest. It isn't a complete victory, but it is nevertheless a shot fired for the cause. I do the wrist-bending, bug-walk thing about twenty more times before my wrist runs out of gas. Movement, any movement, is still a monumental struggle, but the slight improvement I have made today buoys my spirits enough to make me keep trying.

I eventually decide to rest my wrist, and I concentrate instead on the hum and buzz of the hospital waking up. I know I am close to the nurse's station because I can hear people greeting each other and saying their hellos and goodbyes. Shift change is happening. There is much bustling in the morning as the giant machine rumbles to life. Slowly at first, gradually getting louder and up to cruising speed as the morning sneaks away. Mr. Daykin, at twenty-two, has had a rough night, and they have decided to let him sleep. Mr. Johnson is running a temperature blah blah blah. And I'm confident I hear them mention that Mr. Wagner is supposed to be moved today. As if Mr. Wagner needs reminding, mostly because I'm not looking forward to it in the least. It's not that I don't want to have other people around me. I do, but only the people I deem worthy or exciting. I am a selfish patient, and having my own room agrees with me.

The plain but attractive Nurse Chalmers comes in with my breakfast. I'm wondering whether she ever sleeps or gets a day off. Then I realize that I have somehow lost fourteen hours, more than enough time for her to go home and come back. Her hair is held up with a comb of some kind this morning, and she looks fresh and perky as usual. In any other situation I would flirt with her, but unfortunately she has already seen me naked at least a dozen times. The chances of me ever seeing her naked are up there with me teaching a hummingbird to quit flapping its wings and sucking down nectar. So instead of being pleasant and engaging, I opt instead for irritable and cranky.

"I don't want breakfast. The toast is soggy, the coffee is instant, and I stopped eating Red River oatmeal back in the second grade and have no wish to regress."

"Fine, your choice. Did you sleep well?"

"No, I'm afraid to drink the fucking water because sure as shit, a nurse will insist on sticking a rubber hose into the end of my dick."

"Ah, catheters, they are a harsh reality in these trying times. But believe me, the alternative isn't pretty. It's called autonomic dysreflexia."

"Automatic what?"

"No, autonomic. It's called autonomic dysreflexia. It occurs when your bladder backs up. You feel real dizzy and nauseous, you sweat, your heart rate quickens, and then you get sick or you pass out and die. Would you prefer that?"

"Not fucking likely. I'd prefer to stand up and piss like everyone else."

"Not everyone stands up to pee."

"You know what I mean, and why the fuck do I have to move? I'm happy here. Well, relatively happy, but not entirely miserable either. I don't need a whole new battalion of nurses poking and prodding me. So I prefer to go with the Devil-I-know, or something like that."

"A little testy this morning, aren't we? Don't want to move, don't want breakfast."

"You bet; testy, angry, cranky, and pissed off. That's me."

"Good."

"'Good'?" It is not the response I was trying to evoke.

"Anger's healthy. It's part of your little recovery process."

"There you go with the fucking recovery thing again. Weren't you telling me there are five steps? What was it? Denial, which I deny having; anger, how fucking stupid is that step? Like you're supposed to be happy about Quadriplegia; and bargaining, which I further deny having."

"You'll know bargaining when you get to that step."

"So what's the one after bargaining? Assuming I get that far."

She hesitates briefly like this is a crucial step. "Depression," she says reluctantly.

"That's a step? That seems more like a given. Who wouldn't be fucking depressed? These are fucked-up steps. You can't make me believe that some people are tickled pink about losing the use of their arms and legs. Give me a break."

"Depression is different from self-pity. It makes you want to do something about the current situation in which you find yourself. It makes some people try a lot harder to improve. In my experience, I've seen people just get apathetic, and then they lay there like lumps, waiting for some kind of miracle cure instead of improving when and where they can. Basically, they give up. And some people shake it off, talk it out, or look for help."

"Just what I need, a nurse with a minor in psychology. So, what's the fifth step?"

"Acceptance." She apparently likes this step. You can tell by the way she says it.

"Well, I sure as hell haven't arrived at acceptance yet."

"I wouldn't think so. Right now, you're at step two and a half."

"Okay, I'll bite. What's step two and a half?"

"Moving, leaving this private room, and interacting with other patients. It's sandwiched in there somewhere between denial and bargaining. It's a step you can't avoid. You're headed for the seventh floor today, Bub, and it's going to be a bit of a culture shock."

"A 'culture shock', she calls it. I'd call it a giant pain in the ass."

"Call it what you want. It's a reality. You're going to have roommates for the next five to six months, so you might as well get used to it."

"Five to six months? Are you nuts? You can conquer a country in seven months. You could start an empire. Can I get out early for good behavior at four months?"

"Yes, I know, God made Heaven and Earth in seven days. I get your point, but that's just how long this takes; sometimes less, sometimes more. Everyone progresses at their own speed."

"How long what takes? Walking or getting used to laying here?"

"Neither right now. You'll be getting therapy and plenty of it. Therapists will be your best friends and your worst enemies. They will put you to work when you're on the seventh floor—no lollygagging when you're up there. Luckily though, you have to wear the Halo for at least a couple more days. So while you wear the Halo, you are excused from therapy."

"Why does everyone keep saying 'luckily'? I feel anything but lucky, and this Halo contraption itches like crazy."

"So I've heard, but some people wear them for weeks. Hopefully you'll be out of that thing in a couple more days and into a portable. You're lining up even as we speak."

"Bully for me," I say. I'm still not hungry, and the thought of re-entry training makes me want to flip my Red River cereal across the room. I feel capable of great displays of violence, probably because I am completely helpless and have no way to lash out or to emote. As a result, I can't adequately exhibit my frustration. It is a sad day for me. I am not even able to throw Red River cereal. It feels like rock bottom.

"If you're finished with your breakfast, we can get on with the business of moving you. You're going to need another catheterization and then, if you like, we can wait for your family and friends to come back before we take you up to the seventh floor."

"They are way too busy discussing who gets to kill me if I don't improve real soon," I grumble disconsolately. I'm not too fond of the seventh floor because I have no idea what I'm getting into.

"Come again? Who's killing you?"

"Oh, nothing, just thinking aloud. Let's go meet my new roomies, full fucking speed ahead."

"The charge nurse from the seventh floor has to be warned that you're coming, so we can get you all set up."

While she's gone, ostensibly to warn whatever troops they have upon the mysterious seventh floor, two other nurses come in and drain me of precisely 350 milliliters of urine. They immediately rush off to catalog their findings, like little *Keebler Elves*, leaving me alone with my thoughts. I can't help but wonder, and not for the last time, what I have done in this life to deserve the fate that has befallen me.

CHAPTER THIRTEEN

MORE ANGER, ONLY ANGER

MY ENTOURAGE TURNS OUT TO be the pretty but plain, enigmatic, and energetic Nurse Chalmers, along with the charge nurse from the seventh floor, who looks a lot like Margaret Thatcher, only more severe and with longer hair. They are further assisted by a striking blonde nurse who speaks more French than English. I know this because she is constantly muttering to herself in French. I recognize the language from my stay in Cornwall, Ontario, where my wife's bilingual family resides. Her family can swear, sing, and talk all at once in the two official Canadian languages, making a hell of a lot of racket when eight people occupy the same room. I tried to learn the language myself but failed miserably, because who can grasp the intricacies of a language that applies gender specifics to inanimate objects? Why is a table, for instance, feminine, while a pencil is masculine? I could never get beyond that, which ruined my entire French language experience. It's almost as if French people don't want anyone else to learn the language. I am pretty happy to comply.

Nurse Chalmers is thoughtful enough to shoot me up with Demerol before moving me. It is working as near as I can tell because the ceiling panels, which are the same run-of-the-mill drop ceiling panels I have been looking at for days, are suddenly very fascinating. They are wonderfully intricate, graphically designed clouds, but now they move and swirl as the bed rumbles past them. I see the hospital from my back again, and it causes me to wonder, again, why people don't spend more time cleaning the ceiling. It ruins my drug-fueled cloud fantasy. Again, I can see the same old brown watermarks, the same fluorescent plastic light covers where a new army of flies bash themselves against the plastic prison that holds them.

"Why can flies get in there, but they can't get out?" I ask because I am convinced that if somebody can answer that simple question satisfactorily, I will be privy to the secrets of the universe. If I can get inside the mind of just one fly, everything I have done up to this point in my life will become crystal clear. This Demerol is excellent stuff.

"What did he say?" It's the first time the charge nurse has spoken. She sounds all business. Nurse Chalmers answers perfunctorily about my being a little introspective this morning. I sense she doesn't much care for the charge nurse.

"You'll get used to it. Randy is really quite harmless," Nurse Chalmers answers, almost as if she feels the need to defend me.

The French nurse has no comment, so I try to make her understand my query, utilizing my terrible French. "La flies, or le flies as the case might be, ils sont trapped dans la legere. Pourquois?" I'm not sure what she says to this because we have landed in the elevator just as I finish. The good ship Wagner traveling at cruising speed will be coming up to the space dock on the seventh floor. Fasten your seatbelts and return your trays to the upright position.

The doors open, and after I realize the lights up here have their fair share of flies, the smell of the floor engulfs me. It is a sentient being pushing up into my nostrils, infecting my brain, and invading every pore of my body. I can taste it.

"What the fuck is that reek?" I ask. It smells like moldy disinfectant, dirty diapers, and unwashed urinals. This floor would significantly improve with a bit of ventilation or even one barely cracked window. I screw up my nose, which hurts my head and neck, thus allowing my brain a brief respite from the Demerol. "It smells like dead things disguised, but dead things nonetheless."

"You'll get used to it," says the charge nurse. I get the impression they've heard this before, and more than once. It's in the hospital lexicon—right after "be patient."

"It smells like an old folk's home, or at least how I imagine an old folk's home would smell if I had ever visited one. But this isn't the end of the line, is it?" They leave me alone beside the nurse's station, pondering that question while they see to my room assignment. I am left unattended and helpless as they check my bags or whatever they do when you change hospital floors, but I'm not alone for long.

A bleary-eyed, wrinkled old lady, almost bent double at the waist, has come over to inspect me. She does little to dissuade my notion that I have been relocated to the old folk's section of the hospital. She is the walking dead. You can see it in her eyes, the lights have all gone out and the party is long over. She looks me up and down and finds me distasteful somehow because she snorts in disgust and begins to wander away, presumably back to the morgue drawer she crawled out of, leaving room for an even older gentleman to step up. His face is bone thin, and his arms are long and stick-like with hanging flesh and no muscle tone. He sees fit to prod me with his cane, and although I can't feel it, it irks me to no end. It makes the first old woman cackle with glee, prompting him to poke me harder. These morgue people are relentless. I am reliving the "Attack of the Living Morgue People," using canes and cackles instead of their teeth.

"Get fucked, you old coot," I say, hoping to dissuade him with words in place of what I really want to do, which is thump him over the head with his own cane, something I'm not capable of doing at the moment.

"They're just curious," says the plain but pretty Nurse Chalmers, who has come back to my bedside to shoo away the morgue people. "They sit by the elevator all day and wait for family members to visit them. They're bored and alone. It's kind of sad, really."

"Jesus, that is sad," I say, and I can't help but giggle at how silly I sound. Someone sadder than the paralyzed man. Strange times indeed.

"Strokes, Alzheimer's, dementia, senility," she says, slightly shrugging, disregarding the giggling that threatens to overwhelm me. "Their families bring them in and then wait for them to get processed. They're either sent to rest homes or placed in another part of the hospital, the hospice, or—worst-case scenario—they die before they get processed."

"I like this floor a whole bunch already. Tell me more."

"It's a big floor. You'll be with other spinal cord injuries on the west side, but there are a wide variety of illnesses and conditions on this floor. It's predominantly a rehab floor. Most of the people you'll see are here for prolonged physical therapy, and then hopefully, in time, they can get back to their regular lives, and someone picks them up. There are a lot of acute and total care patients just like you."

"Don't call me acute and total care. It makes me sound helpless," but it does get my giggling under control.

"What would you prefer?" she asks.

"I don't know. Is this part of the bargaining step? I don't go in for that politically correct shit, so terms that end in 'challenged' are out. How about 'temporarily fucked up'?"

"Temporarily fucked up it is then. I'll push you down to your room so you can meet some more temporarily fucked up patients like yourself. Your wife is coming, and she'll be here soon, but I'll take you to your room while they process you."

"Don't say processed either. It makes me think of lunch meat or individually wrapped cheese slices."

"Little—"

"Testy?" I finish for her. "You bet I'm a little friggin' testy. This floor ain't exactly Club Med."

"You'll get used to it."

"So I've heard."

"Be patient."

"Bite me." And then she suddenly stops right outside the doorway to the last room on the left. I can only see the top of the door because my head stubbornly refuses to turn sideways—fucking Halo stops that notion. At the end of the large hallway, a sign warns anyone who might want to use the stairwell that an alarm will sound should the door open.

"This is eerie. It's like the *Hotel California*; we are programmed to receive, blah blah blah, but you can never leave, or something like that."

"You can leave anytime you want as soon as you show improvement. Nobody here will try to stop you from walking down those stairs."

"Welcome to the Hotel California, plenty of room at the Hotel California, plenty of fucking rooms at the Hotel California," I start singing. Still, the words don't come easily out of the Demerol fog, so instead I end up repeatedly semi-singing the same part of the song.

"Enough already. Has anyone ever told you that you don't sing well, even for a temporarily fucked up guy?"

"You should have heard me before I broke my neck." I'm not sure exactly what I mean by this, but she laughs all the same. It is an almost sad laugh. I sense that goodbyes are not easy for her. She indeed looks saddened when she explains that I am on my own from here on in. She might be able to pop up and visit, but not often.

Nevertheless, it is a touching moment. In the six (or seven) days I have been in her care, I have come to count on the pretty but plain Nurse Chalmers. She is the only pleasant memory I take from the third floor to the seventh.

"Damn the torpedoes," I say to make light of the situation.

"Damn them all to hell," she says, squeezing my shoulder.

"Oh yeah, and just for the record books, my family and friends aren't planning to kill me." It seems significant that she understands this. I'm hoping it will ease the parting. I'm too stoned to realize how ridiculous my comment sounds, but surprisingly enough she fields this comment well. I think it would be tough to surprise the plain but pretty Nurse Chalmers.

"I know," she says, "I had a chance to talk to your family and friends. They're quite concerned, and the general feeling I got is that they are glad you're still with them. So you're lucky in that regard."

"And disparately unlucky in other regards," and I am left alone with a last squeeze and a smile.

I can hear noises in my new room. It is a sound I can't quite identify. It is a bubbling sound like a kettle that has come to a boil and hasn't been turned off, and someone is playing a Madonna tape, which is not encouraging. Honestly, I'm not too fond of Madonna. And I can smell stale cigarette smoke. I can't decide if it's better or worse than the disinfectant smell, but at least it's recognizable.

Then the Charge Nurse wearing the Margaret Thatcher mask returns, again accompanied by the striking French-speaking blonde nurse and another presence that lurks in the background far enough to be barely noticeable. It appears to be *Doctor Doom*, but I can't be sure until he moves into the room with me and becomes wholly visible for a brief second.

"*Doctor Doom*," I yell as he precedes me into my new digs. Finally, he hears me and reluctantly returns.

"I wish you wouldn't call me that," he says. "It's inappropriate."

"Okay, I'll agree to that. As far as you know, I will never refer to you as *Doctor Doom* again. Are you here to tuck me in?"

"I'm here to get you settled, yes."

"Capital," I say, although I have never used that expression before in my life. The Demerol is making another end-run around my defensive line, sacking my brain. It would be easy to drift off to sleep again, but I will stay awake to make a good impression on my new roommates.

Unfortunately, I can mainly see the ceiling (which I am becoming way too familiar with) as the nurses push me into the room. I can't turn my head very far, and I can only see the semi-curtained-off cubicles where I assume people lie. I am pushed past a bed on each side of me as I make my way to the corner window suite. It is indeed a room with a view.

As I pass by the beds feetfirst on the way to my new home, I am duly informed that the fellow directly to my left and by the door is called Bob. The kettle sound originates from his cubicle, but Bob himself is silent. The percolating sound that I mistook for boiling water is actually air being forced through purified water, which humidifies the air before it gets to Bob's lungs. It is a respirator of some type, but Bob's medical problems don't concern me much.

The fellow across the room, beside the door and right beside the bathroom, is called Wes. He has been here a little over a month, but even as I say, "Howdy, Wes," I am told he is at therapy and will not be back for a while. So I have more or less introduced myself to an empty bed.

The guy in the bed beside Wes, directly across from my feet and in the far corner, is Thomas. But Thomas, much like Wes, doesn't reply when I hail him, albeit for a different reason. He is in a drug-induced coma to keep him quiet and could care less that he has acquired a roommate, and apparently even comatose he enjoys Madonna. Thomas's medical history is briefly described to me. It seems he was riding his bike on the highway, and a passing camper van took him out with the rear-view mirror and then ran over him, breaking several useful bones in both his legs. Even worse, the jolting smack in the back of the head has rendered his brain dysfunctional. The charge nurse reveals this piece of information sotto voce, whispering as if Thomas might wake suddenly should she talk too loudly. There are no secrets on the seventh floor. The French nurse gives me only slightly more insight into the comatose Thomas, addressing me personally for the first time.

"He is not handling it well," she tells me, only she has forgotten to pronounce the H's. Of course, the letter "H" is sheer hell for the French people, but she bravely soldiers on. "He has a head injury also."

"Since 'e is not 'andling 'is 'ead injury well, I suppose I shall 'ave to go easy on 'im," I tell her. I think I'm hilarious, but she doesn't share the moment with me. She remains stone-faced and unimpressed with my accent, so I stop. French people are far too touchy.

The charge nurse and *Doctor Doom* dutifully check me over, and after everything appears hunky-dory, she pulls the curtain between Bob and me. The kettle-on-the-boil sound persists. It is mildly annoying, but I can tune it out with minimal effort. I decide to sleep now and adjust to my new surroundings later.

I quickly take a silent inventory while sleep sneaks up on me. In the far corner is a guy in therapy, to my immediate right is a guy with half a lung, and directly across from me is a guy on heavy-duty drugs with a possible brain injury. Unfortunately, things are not looking up. My roommates have not made an excellent first impression, and I have made no impression on them whatsoever. I promise myself that I will try again later, though, as the move itself has worn me out, and all I want to do is sleep.

I fall asleep before my entourage makes it out of the room, leaving me alone to dream. I dream about being relentlessly pursued by flying monkeys, the same kind that captured Dorothy and pulled the straw out of the scarecrow. When you fall asleep on Demerol, flying monkeys are a relatively everyday occurrence. I had always considered *The Wizard of Oz* a horror story, and this is a horror story. The "monkeys" have arrived.

CHAPTER FOURTEEN

STEP THREE AGAIN: BARGAINING

A LOUD SHRIEKING NOISE BRINGS me out of a fitful slumber. At first, I think that the flying monkeys have somehow followed me out of my dream because what has woken me up can only be described as a banshee-like wail of pain and torment, almost like one of the monkeys is being boiled alive. It continues for a full minute and then stops abruptly, only to continue again after a healthy, noisy intake of breath.

Someone is definitely torturing one of the flying monkeys.

It sounds part animal and part human, and it's coming from directly across the room, where the fellow named Thomas was sleeping so peacefully what seems like mere moments ago. It is not a pleasant sound by any standards. It hurts my brain. I take a deep breath of my own so that I might loudly protest this intrusion, but before I can get the words out, someone speaks for me, taking the terms right out of my mouth.

"Shut the fuck up already," the strange voice yells, louder than I am capable of yelling in my present condition. The strange voice seems to come from across the room and to my right, in the vicinity of where the guy called Wes would be if he were back from therapy. Unfortunately, the curtain the charge nurse has pulled semi-around me surrounds my little area, and I can't see anything save the blue fabric of the curtain. I can hear just fine, though, and as the fellow I assume is Thomas takes another breath and strives to hit all the high notes on the pain scale one more time, I attempt to reason with him along the same lines as the person (who might or might not be named Wes) has done before me.

"Jesus fucking Christ, will you stop screaming!" I implore him.

"He won't listen," says the person who might or might not be Wes. "He wakes up screaming all the time. It's worse at night. If you can walk, why don't you walk over to his bed and smother the dumb fuck with a pillow? I'd pay money to see that."

"I can't walk."

"You must be Randy the Quad then. They said you might be up here soon."

"I've never really thought of myself as Randy the Quad, but I suppose the name is appropriate to the circumstance."

"I'm Wes."

"Wes, what?"

"Wes the Para."

"Funny, but that's not exactly what I meant. What's your last name?"

"Who cares about last names? All that's important is what you are, not who you were. I'm Wes the Para, and you're Randy the Quad to me. I don't give a fuck what your last name is."

"That's a little harsh, don't you think?" I say, wondering what has made this poor soul so negative, but our conversation is cut short by another bout of caterwauling from Thomas, who has cranked up the volume— if that is indeed possible. "Is there any way to shut up Thomas? That is Thomas, I assume?"

"Oh, it's Thomas, all right. Thomas the tard, short for retard, and no, there's no way to shut him up, but it's part of what keeps me going to therapy. One day, when my strength improves, I'll be able to get out of this bed and into a chair, roll the necessary ten feet over to Thomas's bedside, and smother the fuck out of him. I live for that day."

"Weird motivation, dude. What's his problem?"

"Brain injury."

"I was told he's pretty busted up."

"He is, but he's busted up and brain-injured, and it's not a pretty combo. You don't have a fucking brain injury, do you?"

"I haven't ruled out that possibility yet."

"That doesn't sound good. I'd hate to have to smother you too."

"You'd have to get in line." Just as I say this, Thomas shuts up, and there are about thirty seconds of blessed silence before Wes asks me another question, quieter this time. We've both been screaming to be heard above "Thomas the tard," as he has been so unkindly dubbed.

"How long have you been a Quad?" Wes asks.

"Five or six days," I say, not sure exactly what day it is. "About sixty-three catheterizations and two suppositories ago by my reckoning. How about you?"

"One month, about two thousand catheterizations and forty suppositories ago," he says, laughing. I'm greatly relieved that he has a sense of humor. However, I sense it is warped if first impressions carry any weight around this place. Thomas remains mercifully quiet; this is a good thing, because I see spots before my eyes and I'm starting to get dizzy. I'm not very good at shouting over loud noises. I take a few short, shallow breaths to bring my pulse down.

"You still there?" asks Wes, sounding concerned.

"Yeah, I'm still here. Just getting my breath. I couldn't make a career out of screaming over Thomas; I can tell you that."

"You won't have to," he says. "I'm almost to the point where I can get myself out of bed. He'll be dead soon." He says this matter-of-fact-like, as if it is already a foregone conclusion, and I'm beginning to wonder how warped this character might be. I hear what I think is a lighter being flicked.

"You smoking?" I ask.

"You bet," he says. "Pack a day when I can sneak them in. No lectures. Something's going to kill me, and it might as well be cigarettes."

"Heard that before, only it's never sounded more appropriate considering the circumstances. Are you allowed to smoke?" I ask, not caring one way or another as cigarettes have never bothered me overly much. They're dirty stinking things, and I could never imagine myself getting hooked on them. But on the other hand, I drink, and I make no excuses. I've just picked a different poison, and it just happens to be a more socially accept-able route to an early grave.

"Put that out," someone snaps loudly, and my question is answered. Smoking is not allowed.

"Fuck you, Arlene. I will quit smoking when Thomas quits fucking yelling," I hear Wes say right back. It sounds like a fair trade to me. I am willing to *start* smoking if Thomas will stop yelling, and I've just arrived here.

"Put it out, Wes. I'm not going to tell you again." It sounds a little like the charge nurse but with less authority. I sense that even as she's telling Wes that she will not tell him again, she is gearing herself up to tell him as many times as it takes until Wes complies. "It's not what you're doing to Thomas. It's what you're doing to Bob. Bob only has a half of one lung, you know."

"Fuck Bob, nice quality of life, laying there like a goddamn sack of shit hooked to a respirator all day. I'm doing Bob a favor. Right after I smother Thomas, I will do the same to Bob. He'll thank me for it later."

"Don't talk that way. Keep it up and they'll put you in a private room."

"Hah, that's a threat I wish you'd follow up on. Surround me with lunatics and then dangle this private room thing over my head like it's a bad thing. I live for a private room, lady. Well, that, walking again, and getting a blow job from Monique. That little French nurse," he adds loudly, I believe for my benefit.

"A private room with a lock on the door," she counters as the curtains are whisked away, and a nurse I've never laid eyes on before is standing over me. She is built like a girl out of Hugh Hefner's wet dream . . . a five-foot-five playboy model with a smile that goes on forever, large lips, and huge blue eyes you could lose yourself in.

"Hi there," she says. "Don't mind Wes. He's all talk."

"I don't so much mind Wes, but I do mind Thomas. I've been here a couple of hours, and I can already see why Wes might get excited about smothering him. I thought the flying monkeys had followed me out of my dream." Arlene looks at me as if I've lost my marbles, and I hear Wes start laughing until he chokes on his laughter and starts having a coughing fit. He finally puts out his cigarette.

"I like the new guy," Wes manages between hacks. "Finally, someone to talk to. How long you in for?" he asks me.

"Don't know, hopefully not long. It depends on the severity of the injury."

"Yeah, right, and rabbits don't fuck. That's the same shit they peddled to me. It depends on whether it's complete or not. Is your injury complete?"

"I don't think so, although it's hard to say. *Doctor Doom* says . . ."

"Dumars," he corrects me.

"Call him what you want. I call him *Doctor Doom*, like that guy in the *Fantastic Four* comics."

"Say what?"

"Never mind. Anyway, the doc has more or less told me that my chances for a full recovery aren't good, but I could get back ten times more than I have now, which, as it stands, isn't a hell of a lot. Ten times zero is still zero."

"Hey, I hear you, but the first fucking month is always the toughest."

"But I've been told you've only been here a month."

"And it's been the toughest month of my life, let me tell you. Food sucks, it's like they have one pot, and they boil fucking everything, even the Salisbury steaks. And you've met my roommates, but three out of five nurses are pretty hot. Take Arlene, she almost doesn't look old enough to be a nurse, but she looks exotic, a cross between Cher and Angelina Jolie. I am smitten. They don't let the old, fat-assed ones on the seventh floor," continues Wes. "We are labor-intensive, complete-care people. Most of the nurses are kind of friendly. Arlene here has a great set of nuts; she's one of the friendly ones, and she's pretty darn cute." She is all of that.

Arlene blushes and unconsciously holds her hand up in front of what indeed appears to be a "great set of nuts." I decide to let the comment pass, and I question Wes. "You going to get any better?"

"Nope. I'll get stronger, not better. I'm a T-12 Para, which means from about the waist down, I don't feel any more than a dead dog's dick, and I'm complete, so there won't be any sparing."

"A dead dog's dick is not very explanatory. Do your hands work?" I can barely tilt my head enough to see a fuzzy picture of Wes, and he appears to be gripping a trapeze-like device that hangs above his bed. I envy him for the use of his hands already.

"Yeah, but so fucking what? It's from here down that counts." He puts his hand about waist level and swipes downward, taking in the remainder of his prone body. The nurse finally rolls me slightly to the right, sticks pillows under my back, and props the bed up ever so slightly, so I'm getting my first honest good look at Wes. He has a hawk-like face framed by a huge mass of unruly, unkempt, streaked blond hair that would be more at home gracing the head of either a rock star or a bag lady. He is emaciated, but ropy ridges of muscle stand out on his skinny arms as he grasps his trapeze and shifts his bony ass over an inch or two. He still has the snubbed-out cigarette in his mouth, and he looks world-weary. Too world-weary for his age, as I judge him to be all of thirty years old, give or take, about the same age as me, but he could easily pass for fifty. He looks like Mick Jagger's younger brother.

"How old are you?" I ask him.

"Thirty-four, going on sixty," he tells me, more or less confirming what I had already guessed.

"What happened to you?" I ask. People's prognoses suddenly seem essential. I am trying to relate to Wes, but I can't get past *his* hands working while mine lie dormant. It is the first time I think that all injuries are relative. While I envy something as simple as using his hands, which I had previously taken for granted, he aspires to the next level. Since he already has his hands, he can now concentrate on using his legs, while I will gladly settle for opposable thumbs.

"I jumped out of a tree," Wes informs me.

"That broke your back?"

"Nope. I landed on a truck."

"And that broke your back?"

"Nope, then the truck ran over me."

"I'm almost afraid to ask. What happens next?"

"And that's when I broke my back."

"Good story—fucking complicated, but better than mine."

"I was dead-ass drunk."

"I would hope so, unless this whole jumping out of trees into trucks is an Alberta pastime?"

"We were way out in the boonies. They had to drive me to the hospital in the back of the truck. Who knows what might have happened if my three friends had called an ambulance."

"What do you mean?"

"It gets worse if someone moves you. Did somebody move you?"

"A little, I guess." I take a moment then and think back. I had been moved, but it never occurred to me that moving me might have added to my injury. I distinctly remember the smell of gas, and I vaguely recall that my wife was afraid the truck would blow up. How far had she moved me? I really couldn't say. Had my neck flopped around like one of those spring-loaded nodding dogs that sit on the back windows of mobster cars? I had no clue. It was something I didn't even want to consider. What's done is done. Wishes are not horses, and I wouldn't be riding out of here soon. Going over the possibilities would get me nowhere quickly, and I would never ask these questions out loud. Truth be known, I didn't want to hear the answers.

Wes is strangely quiet, busy rehashing his injury as if he was reading my thoughts, but the moment gets lost as Adams, Bignell, and Shea come into the room. My mother, wife, and aunt aren't far behind.

"Nice room," says Shea sarcastically, taking in the surroundings and delivering the verdict without the benefit of a trial. The others take up the ball where Shea has dropped it.

"Yeah, nice. Who did you piss off?" asks Bignell.

"Same hotel, same price, but with snazzy blue curtains and room-mates," I add needlessly. "I'm moving up in the world, but enough with the room already. That guy over there is Wes," I say, staring at Wes needlessly because he is only twelve feet away and quite obviously the only one up for an introduction. "This guy on my right is Bob. He has half a lung, and the percolating sound you hear is Bob's respirator, which I understand subs in for Bob's lungs when they tire out, or it gives him moisture in his lungs so they don't clog up or something like that. He has what Wes here calls no quality of life. The guy across the way is Thomas. He has a head injury and can make more noise than a damned scalded cat. As of this moment, that is all I know about him. Try not to wake him up or piss him off. For that matter, don't do anything that might startle him and make him start screaming again."

"I plan to smother him," Wes announces. Obviously, he is the worst smotherer in history because this seems to be his goal in life, and he is not good at it. With that thought, Wes lights a cigarette and pretends to ignore us.

My family and friends look around the room, digesting. They are not impressed, but they will try to put a good spin on the situation. I'm curious as to how this might be possible.

"Could be worse," my wife says on cue, ever polite and cheerful. Wes says a "pleased to meet you" and then instructs Arlene (with the great nuts) to shut his curtain so we can have some privacy. I almost laugh at this, but I understand the gesture, so I keep quiet. The idea that a thin blue curtain will give anyone privacy is comical, but it is the only form of privacy available. It is another grim prospect. Especially to someone like me who prioritizes solitude, but it is something I will have to deal with later as my friends and family look uncomfortable. It is my job to maintain morale.

We talk about inanities for an hour or so, which puts them more at ease. I'm sure they didn't expect me to make a miraculous recovery during the night, but the way they are having trouble looking me in the eye is disconcerting. The gradual healing process I am doomed to go through will be arduous for them. Convalescing in Calgary, far away from close friends and family, might be the best for everybody. It is not the first time I have considered this.

As if reading my mind, my mother puts voice to my concern. "We've talked to the doctor and a very informative social worker here at the hospital, and they both think it might be a good idea for you to fly back to the Vancouver area when your bones straighten up and you're stable. They've got a great hospital there just for people who have spinal cord injuries, and it is a lot closer to home. It's called GF Strong."

"Nice name," I say, not yet willing to share my reluctance to recuperate close to people who would be inclined to monitor my every move. "Let's cross that bridge when we come to it." The look of relief on my wife's face after my comment is painfully apparent, and I am glad she is at the back of the receiving line and out of sight of my mother. I can relate to her.

The bottom line is that we have a restaurant to open up in Calgary—well, Airdrie. Though this might seem like a minor distinction to my family considering the injuries I've sustained, it is still my wife's dream come true, and any delay would destroy her. She has waited for this opportunity for what probably seems like three forevers put together. I have also been considering our responsibilities to our partners while I've been lying here, and as I see it we only have one option. I will have to recover as much as I can as quickly as I can and do it in the Calgary General Hospital so the restaurant opening will not be delayed. I will slowly break this idea to my mother.

Arlene is in the background now, holding up her wrist and glancing at her watch. I don't know whether she is telling me that it's time for drugs or a catheter. I don't much care either way. By this time, we have exhausted all possible avenues of what I have come to think of as cheery hospital chatter, and I'm getting tired. Ideally, in a hospital situation, visitors would come one at a time and stay for about eight minutes before disappearing to make way for the next ones. Arlene assures me this will only take about ten minutes—it is a catheter, after all—but my friends need a break as much as I do. They want to get stinking drunk and talk about why their friend Randy Wagner is fucked up and may never walk again. They don't understand *paralyzed* yet, and they want to discuss it over a cold one. They are all secretly glad it's me and not one of them laying here, and I don't blame them. If I were in their place, I would think the same thing.

They take my mother with them, but my wife stays behind because she wants to understand how to catheterize a Quadriplegic. I am secretly pleased that not everyone shares her curiosity.

Nurse Arlene doesn't even ask me whether I am the least bit uncomfortable with someone else in the room. She assumes that my wife will have to know this procedure in the future, and she is only too happy to play instructor. So I watch as if from a great distance. First, she shows my wife how to swab the end of my dick with an alcohol swab, allowing her to do it too, and then she inserts the catheter after greasing up the end of it with gel. My wife also helps her with this stage of the performance, and they are doing some heavy-duty organ manipulation—tag-teaming—passing my dick back and forth like a relay baton, and I get an unscheduled surprise hard-on. Big surprise because it's not as if I can feel what they are doing, and getting a catheter stuffed into the head of your dick and fed down to your bladder is certainly not, in any way, sexually exciting. But there it is, pretty as you please, demanding attention, like a first grader standing up in the middle of the class waving his hands and shouting, "Oooh, oooh, pick me."

I try to pretend it isn't happening, but my wife will not let the moment pass.

"Wag, you've got a hard-on," she says unnecessarily.

"It's pretty common," says Arlene, entirely at ease, "The stimulation causes an autonomic reaction. He can't help it, and he can't prevent it."

"That's weird," says my wife, echoing my thoughts exactly. I can barely hear giggling about eleven or twelve feet away through two privacy curtains. Wes hears everything being discussed. Privacy curtains, my ass. My bladder is draining far too slowly for my liking.

"Shut the fuck up, Wes," I say, bewildered but curious about this new occurrence. Behind the privacy curtain, we are all staring at my erection as if it alone can illuminate why it should suddenly and inexplicably appear. "Is this going to happen all the time?" I ask Arlene.

"No. As I was saying to your wife, it's called an autonomic erection. You have no control over it. Perhaps I should let your doctor explain, but it's pretty simple. Direct stimulation causes a reaction you have no control over, any more than you could control the beating of your heart or the working of your lungs. Sometimes it happens just because the temperature of the room changes or you have a spasm attack."

"So I could get an erection at any time? It's like being fourteen again." I am digesting the ramifications of this new revelation, if that is what it is.

"Only when you don't want one," says Wes. Since he seems so determined not to be excluded from the conversation, I speak to him directly.

"So what's the deal, Wes? I can get a woody at any time, day or night?" I am still uncertain whether this is a good thing or a bad thing.

"Yep," says Wes. "Problem is, they're relatively useless, like having a gun with no bullets. Like having a bottle of champagne and no . . ."

"I read you just fine here, Wes," I interrupt, and as if on cue, my hard-on dissipates slowly as Arlene flicks it very hard with her pointing finger. It is scared back into unconsciousness, afraid of the spotlight. I look at my wife, and she shrugs her shoulders. We are both bewildered, but the questions will come later when the audience goes home and we have more time and absolute privacy. Arlene senses this and hurriedly but efficiently extracts the catheter, cleans up after herself, and exits without exchanging another word. Now it is my turn to shrug. Only when I try, my head turns slightly, and I feel a sharp twinge of pain shoot up my neck, causing me to grimace before I can stop myself.

"You okay, Wag?" asks my wife, noticing my discomfort and probably glad to focus on something else besides unscheduled hard-ons.

"Yeah, nothing a brand-new spinal cord wouldn't fix," I say, grinning stupidly, causing my wife's eyes to tear up. It seems all of my attempts at dry humor are destined to fall flat, and it makes me wonder whether there might ever come a time when we can laugh about this. "I'm just a little tired," I add, refusing to succumb to self-pity. "Why don't you go catch up with the rest of the crew and drink a few cold pops for me? A nurse should be along anyway to shoot me up with drugs and wrestle me back onto my left side. I'll see everyone later on."

"Are you sure?"

"I'm sure," I say, wishing to be left alone more than anything. I am tired, but more than that, my mind is racing with unanswered questions. My wife finally leaves after assuring me that she will be back soon, and I hear Wes light up another cigarette as soon as she goes, so I know he is still awake.

"Okay, Wes, humor me. I'm a rookie at this, but what's with the automatic hard-on?" I ask him.

"Autonomic, not automatic," he corrects me. "It's a tease is what it is, it pops up when you least expect it, and it doesn't serve any real purpose . . . Are you sure you want to hear this shit? Hell, you might recover more than you expect. But don't sell yourself down the river yet. Quads get 'em more than Paras."

"Just keeping current, Wes, don't worry about me. I'm an information sponge. So, tell me what Nurse Arlene was talking about when she mentioned spasm attacks. Just what the hell is a spasm attack?"

"Oh, you picked up on that, did you? It's another thing Quads get. Paras don't get them as much. It's like your body gets an electric shock or something. Carl could tell you more. He lives two doors down and has been here for two months or even a little longer. He's a Quad just like you, only he's got no fucking sense of humor at all, refuses even to try therapy, and he's a real prick to talk to."

"Can't wait to meet him. If you happen to run into him, tell him to visit me if he's got a chance. I've got a lot of questions."

"'If he's got a chance.' Jesus Christ, Rook, listen to yourself. Do you think we got a lot to do around here? Someone new on the floor is like a happening. He already knows you're here."

"What do you do around here, now that you mention it?"

"Smoke cigarettes and joints, drink free pop and coffee, watch T.V., have little fantasy circle jerks over the few decent looking nurses, you know, just normal spinal cord injury shit. Most of the people in here are what you might call institutionalized."

"That ain't for me, partner. It'll be a cold fucking day in hell before I get institutionalized. What about therapy? What's that like?"

"Sucks, but it breaks up your day. They wake you up around seven or eight, then force-feed you the cream of fucking wheat, oatmeal, or Red River cereal, and after that they send you down to the pit where trained therapists make you jump through hoops till you get so fucking tired you'll want to puke. Then, after all the fun is over, you come back upstairs for a delicious Wonder Bread cheese sandwich and a fruit cup for lunch, and then you take a well-deserved nap."

"I don't nap," says the guy who has done nothing but for the last five— or is it six—days.

"You'll learn. After that, if you're lucky you get into a wheelchair and make someone push you outside if you can't do it yourself, where you can breathe real air and there are no fucking screaming retards and mummi-fied older people. Then it's suppertime. They feed the zoo animals first, in the lounge, but you get to eat in your room, which is a real break. Whatever you do, make damn sure they feed you in your room. It's fucking gross watching the Raisins eat. After supper, you go up to the roof on the eighth floor, smoke a big fat joint, and then you go to bed while the rest of the world parties, fucks, drinks, and dances."

"You got this pretty well mapped out."

"You bet."

"No forks in the road, no speed bumps, no glitches?"

"Oh, you'll get glitches; you'll get glitches up the ass. I'm just giving you a best-case scenario. In the hospital, boring is good."

"That was a best-case scenario. So what's a worst-case scenario?"

"You don't want to know."

"You're probably dead right on that one. What about visitors?"

"What about 'em?"

"They must fit in somewhere."

"Fuck visitors, that's enough with the questions anyway. You ask a lot of fucking questions. Get some sleep while you can. Thomas doesn't shut up just because it's dark out. Do you want your drugs? I can pull the ripcord."

"The what?"

"Ripcord, that string behind your head. It lights up a panel just outside the room and sounds an alarm at the nursing station. Sends the nurses scrambling. Can you reach yours?"

"Reach it? I can't even see it," but I sense this is an essential tool.

"You'll have to get that fixed up. That's your lifeline. Tell you what, just ask me if I'm here, and I'll do the pulling for now, but you'll need a ripcord of your very own. A ripcord is power around here." Wes must have pulled the ripcord because a nurse came into the room only minutes later, and she pulled Wes's curtain open. He directed them to me, and I got my drugs, and all was well.

At least until Thomas woke up again.

CHAPTER FIFTEEN

ANGER AND
BARGAINING PERSIST

AT LEAST THIS TIME I'M not dreaming about flying monkeys picking my body apart when Thomas chooses to put a voice to his inner terrors. No, this time I am dreaming about floating. I'm above the treetops, and I can see the house where I grew up, and I can't figure out what I'm doing back there. I am right in the middle of landing in my old backyard when Thomas sounds off. It screws up my landing, and I fall to Earth real quick. At first, I thought it was the hospital smoke detector, a backup alarm on a dump truck, or a car alarm.

"YOOOOWEEE, YOOOWEEE," yells Thomas at previously undocumented volumes. Kind of like a general call to arms in a submarine, only much louder.

"YAAAAEEEEYAAA," he continues, switching mid-yell to a police siren sound. I know I would be inclined to pull over very quickly if I had been driving at this particular moment. I cannot imagine being rudely awakened like this every time I dream, be it good or bad.

"Pull the ripcord," I yell over to Wes, hoping like hell that he's awake, although if he's here, he's bound to be awake.

"I already pulled it," he yells back.

"Pull it again."

"You can only pull it once. After that, just stick your fingers in your ears."

"Funny fucking guy, Wes."

"Oh, yeah, sorry about that."

"Hey Wes, tell me again how you plan to smother Thomas," I say, emphasizing the smothering part, drawing it out as if saying it loud enough might make it spontaneously happen. And even as I get the words out of my mouth, Thomas abruptly clams up. His voice still echoes in the sudden silence, but the cacophony has ceased. I'm unconsciously biting my lip, bracing for the next round, but nothing happens. I can almost hear Wes holding his breath across the room, but the only sound is the constantly boiling kettle signifying Bob's tenuous hold on life, and it's boiling heavily right now. Thomas has upset Bob, if that is at all possible.

"You think he heard me?" I ask Wes.

"Who? Bob?"

"No, idiot. Thomas."

"Not fucking likely. I've been yelling at him for two weeks now, and I've never gotten any response."

"Hey, Thomas!" I yell. "Can you hear me?" Unfortunately, hospitals play havoc with your mind, and though I no longer intend to smother him now that he has ceased caterwauling, the idea that I wanted to gnaws at my conscience a little bit. I get no response, so I try again. "Hey, Thomas, if you can hear me or understand me, say something. Start yelling again if that's all you can do."

"Fuck you, too," says Wes.

"Speak to me, Thomas," I say, ignoring Wes. I'm convinced that Thomas is aware more than ever, and my efforts are rewarded when I hear a voice right from where Thomas would be.

"T-T-T-Thomas," the voice stutters.

"Holy shit," says Wes.

"T-T-T-Thomas TEE T-T-Thomas," the voice says, and then again, only louder. "T-T-T-Thomas TEE T-T-Thomas, T-T-THOMAS TEE T-T-THOMAS, TEE-TEE-TEE T-T-THOMAS T-T-T-THOMAS." Then, finally, the voice crescendos to match Thomas's previously reserved volume for wailing. "T-T-T-THOMAS!" the voice delights over and over again.

"Oh, fucking terrific. Way to go, mister fucking concern. Tell him to go back to just plain yelling," says Wes.

But the nurse has arrived by now, and she seems pretty excited about this new development. It is a new nurse—at least new to me—and she asks Wes right away how long Thomas has been speaking.

"Too fucking long," answers Wes, not sharing her excitement. "If you can call what he's doing speaking."

"He just started," I say. "He was yelling, and then he stopped right after I suggested that Wes smother—uh, right after Wes pulled the cord. Has he ever talked before?"

"Nope, this is the first time. He's been completely unresponsive up to now, except for the yelling," she informs me.

Meanwhile, Thomas is still stuttering his name at half volume. He seems pretty pleased with just saying his name repeatedly, while the new nurse and I are content just to listen. Wes, however, is not and expresses his displeasure.

"We're all really fucking happy that Thomas can say his name, but before we continue this conversation, would you mind sticking a balled-up sock in his yap. He's driving me fucking crazy. Some of us like to sleep at night."

"Always the sentimentalist, hey, Wes?" says the nurse, but she comforts Thomas with gentle words, calming him down. She asks him some simple questions, but she gets no response. He is still repeating the same thing, "Thomas T-Thomas," but quietly now, like a mantra. Compared to the howling he is capable of, this is a godsend. The new nurse talks to him a bit longer, and his litany is reduced to a whisper before she disengages herself and comes through the privacy curtain to the side of my bed.

"Hello," she says, whispering, which is quite comical given the circumstances. She is certainly in no danger of waking anyone up at this point, but somehow her whispering is soothing. Even Bob's kettle is simmering on low, so I follow her lead.

"Hello," I whispered right back. "And who might you be?"

"Pam," she says. "And you're Randy, right? Your wife and some friends were here around seven-thirty, but they said not to wake you. They'll be back to see you tomorrow."

Pam asks me a batch of questions: how am I feeling, do I need anything, and would I like to be repositioned? She has a quiet confidence, an air about her that lets you know she is genuinely concerned, and it's not faked or contrived. I believe this is a nurse thing. The French nurse has it, as does the pretty but plain Nurse Chalmers, who has it in spades. It's almost as if they understand what you're going through, and they truly care but don't feel pity for you. I'm left with the impression that they are there to help without reservation or question.

Pam has just started her rotation of four night-time shifts in a row. She offers to get me something to eat because I have slept through supper and my last turn, which I find kind of strange since I've never slept through a turn before that I can recall. I have been out of it for some time because it is dark outside, and it's late, although how much time has passed is a mystery. I think once more how time seems so immaterial in the situation I'm in. One day just rolls into the next. I have given myself over to their care, and few events are separating the days behind me or, I suspect, the days ahead of me.

I take a quick inventory by rote, it's something I do now without thinking, and nothing seems to have changed. I feel groggy, thirsty, and sweltering, but my limbs are as immobile and unresponsive as they were the last time I checked.

Pam offers me water, and I suck about a gallon of it through the tiny straw before I'm satisfied. It's then that she notices I've been sweating. The sheets are soaked, and my forehead is on fire. Not just cause for immediate alarm, but Pam switches on the lights anyway to check me out more thoroughly.

"What now?" says an exasperated Wes. "This is turning into one hell of a night."

"Randy's running a small fever," says Pam. It seems there are no secrets in this room. If I'm burning up with a fever, then Wes must be duly informed.

"Check him for clots," says Wes, suddenly awake and animated.

"You don't check for clots, Wes," Pam tells him. "You check for swelling."

"Swelling, clots, same fucking thing," says Wes, and while this conversation is taking place, Pam has rolled me over on my side and has flipped the sheet off of me. Pam is efficient, and there is no wasted motion. She is sure of herself, the consummate professional, belied only by wild red hair, multiple piercings, and tattoos. So while checking me out, I am doing the same to her. A petite, compact, very sexy lady, with all the curves where they should be and the couple extra pounds she carries fill her out more in all the right places. About thirty-five, tough-looking, but a person you can feel comfortable with from the first minute you meet her. She has five earrings or more in one ear and another half dozen or so in the other. There is a tattoo just below her earlobe of a teardrop. Another tattoo peeks up just above her collar, and there is just enough revealed to hint that there might be a mural under her shirt. I see what I think might be an eagle. It almost makes me forget what she is searching for—well, almost.

"What's a blood clot?" I ask, not alarmed but beginning to feel mildly nauseous. Anything that gets Wes animated can't be a good thing.

"Silent killers," says Wes. "Little ninjas that come in the night and clog up your arteries." He is doing nothing to allay my fears, filling me chock-full of what he considers pertinent information.

"That's enough, Wes," says Pam.

"No, it's not," I say, more than mildly intrigued. "What are you talking about, Wes?"

"Blood clots, man. They break off and head straight for your heart or your brain, and 'Wham! Bam! Thank You, Ma'am!' you're dead before you can scream."

"Shut up, Wes," says Pam. At the same time, she's busy comparing my left calf to my right, holding both up and looking at them curiously, although it's obvious even to me that the left is larger and more swollen than the right. This is because the skin of the left calf is taut and bloated.

"The left calf's swollen," I say unnecessarily.

"Bingo, fucking blood clot," says Wes triumphantly, clapping his hands together like he's just answered a True Daily Double on *Jeopardy*.

"Might be," says Pam, "but it ain't no big deal. It'll keep till morning, and we'll check it out then."

"If you live that long, Quad-Boy," says Wes, enjoying himself. I'm now quite certain that Wes is a trifle more screwed up than I initially believed. Through his simple harmless outbursts and mordant lousy humor, he seems to derive some kind of vicarious pleasure from everyone else's misery. Pam thinks much the same as I do.

"Fuck you, Wes, and for the last time, shut up, or you might find yourself getting a high colonic with a hot poker in about ten seconds." I decide I like Pam a lot. After dealing with Wes, she turns back to me, and her bedside manner becomes professional once more.

"We'll take your temperature and blood pressure and increase your Heparin drip, but there's no reason to panic. Contrary to popular belief, blood clots do not break up and head straight for your heart or brain, at least not if they're treated. Anyone with a spinal cord injury is prone to blood clots. They aren't rare, and they are even expected in most cases. They were a cause for concern twenty years ago, but now they are very treatable. The worst that can happen is that we put you on a clot machine in the morning and check if it is indeed a blood clot."

"Warfarin," pipes up Wes.

"Warfarin, Heparin, they're different names for the same drug. Basically, it's a blood thinner," explains Pam.

"It's fucking rat poison," says Wes, clearly not fearful of a high colonic, whatever that might be. "Call it whatever fancy name you want. But in the end, it all spells goddamn rat poison." But, of course, he is needlessly pointing out the things I know.

Pam maintains eye contact with me, and she makes a circle around her left ear—which has more like ten earrings in it on closer inspection—signifying that Wes is quite loopy and is not to be taken too seriously. I know she is trying to reassure me, and it works to some degree. I sense that she wants to tell me more, but it will have to wait for another time because Thomas has begun to pick up the chant again. Now that he has regained the power of speech—if it can be called chanting—he seems determined not to let it lapse again. Pam makes do with a tired smile and a shrug, conveying both her concern for me and her helplessness to control the situation. She reaches over and pulls the ripcord above my head and goes back to Thomas's bedside, calming him down with kind words and deft touches. He has drifted off to sleep before the French nurse Pam has summoned arrives, and then I become their primary focus. Together they take my temperature and my blood pressure, and I am deemed fit enough to survive the night without any interference save my usual shot of Demerol and an extra helping of Heparin for good measure.

I'm left alone after that to reflect on my first day up on the seventh floor, and I see how far I have fallen in the short time I have been here. I'm convinced I'm not getting better; I'm getting worse. My head feels like it's being extricated from my shoulders, and their added weight makes it even worse. I just wish my goddamn bones would line up so we can get on with it. Then I can get my operation and maybe a more detailed explanation of my future well-being. At this point, I will think happy thoughts if I can walk again. Even *Pinocchio* had a do-over.

CHAPTER SIXTEEN

BACK TO DENIAL AND MORE ANGER

AMAZING WHAT A GOOD NIGHT'S drug-induced slumber can do for you. The morning finds me in high spirits. I have been inspected early this morning, and my left calf is swollen and distended, so I have been put on a machine designed specifically to diagnose blood clots, and it comes as no surprise to anyone that I do indeed have one. The nurses assure me that this is common and should be taken in stride, so I attempt to do just that.

It does prompt a visit from *Doctor Doom*. They crank up the volume on the Heparin drip, just another bag of mystery liquid and a new I.V. pole. It is totally different than Peter Pole. The new one has a computer array, and it beeps every now and then. *Doctor Doom* tells me this will set my operation back indefinitely, but I don't care. I don't care because I can lift my arm off the bed.

Not a whole lot, but it is a huge victory, nonetheless.

I imagine I can feel the power flowing back into my body. I'm even half convinced that I will be walking soon. I know it is silly and perhaps even dangerous to think in these terms in the back of my mind, but I need a lift. If Wes were not already down in therapy, I would tell him about this new development. Instead, I decided to share my thoughts with Thomas T. Thomas, who has now taken to calling himself this regularly to anyone who will listen. Thomas has slept through the night and has woken up with the conviction that this is his name, and no amount of convincing to the contrary shall shake this belief. He has pointed to himself no less than forty times, repeating his name with a sense of certainty that invites challenge. I have no desire to challenge his assertion.

My bed has been propped up, and I can see Thomas. He has a thin face with a crooked smile and a small mustache. I don't think he could grow a full one. He is young. Twenty-five is my rough guess. His shoulders are broad, but the rest of him is emaciated—do they not feed people on the seventh floor? He looks military, with closely cropped hair with a prominent brow, and his eyes look crazed. No surprise there.

I had once heard that it's easier to unburden your deepest fears and concerns with a total stranger than with someone close to you, and I am going to test this hypothesis. I have no fear of reprisal because Thomas is not about to shout my deepest fears and concerns from every rooftop.

"Thomas," I begin, but he makes an unintelligible sound before I can continue.

"AACCKK," he says, in such a way as to leave little doubt something is amiss.

"Thomas," I begin again.

"AAACCKK," he says again, and he points to himself. Again, I feel like a fool. What could I have been thinking?

"Thomas T. Thomas," I say, and he beams with pride. "I am at a crossroads here. I believe my family and friends want me to heal in Vancouver, which is closer to the happy home front, but I think this would be the wrong way to go. Okay, on the plus side, I'll get more visitors, but I might not dedicate enough time to therapy. I'll have support, but it will be smothering. You know what I mean?" Thomas stares at me like I'm reciting from tablets brought fresh from Mount Sinai that morning, so I decide to keep rambling.

"I've got a restaurant to open, damn it, and I have to focus on that. We've come a long way to get to this point, and I have to think of my wife. She fits into the big picture somewhere, and I wouldn't have gotten this far without her. But, and this is where it gets confusing, Tom. Can I call you Tom?"

"AACK," he says and cocks his head sideways like a bird.

"Thomas T. Thomas it is then. No matter, it's just that I've never told anyone this before, but if the truth is known, I never really wanted to open a restaurant. So there, I said it. You'll never know how tough that was. But that's not the whole truth either. So let me start at the beginning."

I take a deep breath because it's hard to speak for any length of time, and I briefly rest before I start again. The look on Thomas T. Thomas's face lets me know he's still partially with me. His eyes have never left my face. Now that I think about it, I haven't seen him blink for five minutes. When I don't continue immediately, he waves his hands around, and finally he points to himself once more, and then he points at me. It's like conversing with Tarzan.

"Thomas," he says, and it's all the prompting I need. He has the smile of a first grader spelling a three-letter word correctly for the first time. "Thomas," he says again needlessly.

"Thomas works for me, guy. Anyway, Thomas, it's my wife's dream, not mine. It's just that I don't truly have a dream of my own, so I'm sharing hers, and I thought that would be enough, but it isn't. I mean, opening our restaurant is great, and it's way better than a real job where you punch a clock, but it isn't going to be easy. I spent my entire life taking the easy road, and this might be more than I can handle. Maybe that's it. I'm afraid of failure."

Thomas is still with me, I think. He's staring wide-eyed right at me, and it's enough to keep me going now that I've started. "Maybe that's why I never gave myself over to one single thing entirely. That way I never had to see it right to the end. You know what I mean?"

Thomas finally blinks, but he still looks at me quizzically, at least somewhat aware, and I'm unsure whether to continue. The untimely arrival of Wes, who is back from therapy, takes away all doubts. I have no desire to share my inner thoughts with Wes, the sarcastic and myopic misery vampire. When Wes enters, I shut up, and Thomas immediately becomes agitated. He lets out a couple of war whoops that would not have been out of place at the Little Big Horn. All the time, he is staring at Wes, shooting what could only be called invisible hate darts and death rays from his eyes.

"What are you gawking at, Tard-Boy?" Wes asks, and it prompts Thomas to point at himself for the umpteenth time that morning.

"Thomas T. Thomas," he tells Wes, a little adamantly.

"Yeah, I know. I fucking heard you last night. Thomas 'T' for Twit Thomas."

"AACCKK," says Thomas, clearly perturbed at Wes.

"AAACCKK yourself, fuckhead," says Wes, who looks exhausted. Therapy has drained him, and he seems relieved when a nurse comes in to help him into his bed. His exchange with Thomas is forgotten until Wes is ready to transfer into his bed.

"Watch this, Thomas Tard Thomas. I can pretty well get to bed by myself. I just need a little help with my legs. Do you know what that means? It means that since I can almost get into bed by myself, I can *also* almost get out of bed by myself, which puts me that much closer to the day when I can fucking smother your ass in your goddamn sleep."

This commentary brings on another round of war whoops and the usual remonstrations from the nurse of the day. She is big, with plump cheeks and a prominent forehead because her hair is receding. She introduces herself to me, and I say hello, but her name doesn't stick in my brain. I could have met her yesterday, for all I know. She is Filipino, however, which sets her apart from the others. Her English is not very good, but adequate for the job at hand.

"You shut you fat mouth, Wesley. You not help, you keep quiet," she says, and I'm inclined to agree with her.

"Yeah, you not help, shut you fat mouth, Wesley," I mimic unnecessarily. Wes grumbles a reply I don't quite catch, although it sounds suspiciously like a racial slur, which is about what I'd expect from him. It causes the Filipino nurse to drop his legs unceremoniously on the bed, leaving the final stage of the transfer to him.

"Besides, it's much better to have an awake Thomas than the screaming blue murder coma-version you're used to," I continue, trying to lighten up the sudden tension in the room. Still, I can feel Wes's anger and frustration, almost like a physical presence. My day is not nearly as rosy as it first appeared to be. Moods are so fickle in a hospital environment. Yessiree, there's nothing like a damn hospital and dysfunctional roommates to

remind you that you're physically decrepit. So I decided to go for another opinion. "What do you think, Bob? Just gurgle once for yes, twice for no."

"You no help either you," says the Filipino nurse, whose nametag announces that she would like to be called Althuna, once I take the trouble to read it. "Bob, he hear every word. He understand everything."

"Sure he does, Al-tuna," Wes says. "Bob here doesn't miss a fucking trick. Do you, Bob?"

"Althuna," she says patiently, making her name sound almost musical and breathy, unlike Wes's pronunciation, which pegged her as a species of fish with a first name.

"Whatever you say, I'll call you Al," dismissing her like an asshole. Wes is responsible for altering my good humor, and I should have taken it out on him, but the strange thing is that I can't bring myself to pick on a cripple, no matter how contrary he gets. He has more movement or "sparing" than I have, but I haven't yet categorically come down to his level. More denial? Maybe, but it is still too early to start pigeonholing my condition. I can't even say the word cripple out loud, let alone classify myself as one of their numbers.

"How'd therapy go, Wes?" I ask, not yet willing to completely surrender my good mood. Maybe if I can cheer Wes up, I can turn my mood around.

"Great, I batted balloons around to improve my balance and tried to roll over several times with some success. After that, I went to the head of the fucking class. I got a gold star and a reminder that I'm pretty well fucking useless. Anything else you want to know?"

"Nope," I say, abandoning any hope of revitalizing my good mood. Instead, I'm glad when Althuna pulls his privacy curtain shut and he goes into nap mode.

I go into the same mode because I have very little else to do. My neck is fucking killing me slowly, and I have lost the urge to talk to Thomas. And as for old one-lung Bob, he may understand what I'm saying, but he is still a mystery to me and not someone I'm apt to confide in. Since my arrival, he has been wearing a face mask, and unless he shows more signs of life, it is easier to ignore him. Even Darth Vader was more communicative and slightly less noisy.

CHAPTER SEVENTEEN

STEP FOUR: DEPRESSION, FINALLY

DAY THIRTY-THREE. THIRTY-THREE OF THE longest days of my life, and a lot has changed. Bob is dead. He died during the night. He didn't so much die as he just ceased to make noise. One minute his kettle was merrily boiling along, and then the next minute it was deathly silent, literally and figuratively.

They wheeled him out in the early hours. There is no fanfare or final hurrah, just a straight blip on a monitor, and the Bob I never knew is gone. It makes me feel fragile and lonely. It makes me feel inconsequential, like I could die during the night and nobody would notice. But on the other hand, I suddenly want people around me.

My friends, my mother, and my Aunt Dorene have all gone. They all stayed about one week, and after failing to convince me that recuperating closer to home would be in my best interests, they departed to let me fight the good fight on my terms.

My mother left with a heavy heart, and my friends left confused. I was confused because they couldn't quite grasp what was wrong with their old buddy Wagner. I looked healthy enough. Sure, I'd lost a lot of weight, but what was holding up my recovery? I secretly think my buddies were glad

I picked Calgary as my institution of choice. Unfortunately, they will be in denial a lot longer than I will.

Wes gets better every day. His strength has improved dramatically, and he is up and pushing around almost at will. He has mastered the all-important transfer from bed to chair. I envy him. I have not made great strides myself.

After my right arm moved, I peaked for a while and felt quite discouraged. But there have been some improvements, but anything short of kicking a field goal is considered little progress by my way of thinking. My left arm has regained partial movement, making it only slightly less useless than the other one, so now I can spider-walk both my hands up to my face to scratch my nose if I can find it. Unfortunately, my fingers are still useless. So I essentially have paws, curled-up paws. My clenched fists look like I'm ready to scrap, but nothing could be farther from the truth.

I have not been granted the opposable thumb option that sets humans apart from animals and puts us slightly higher up on the food chain. In short, I can't grip sweet fuck all, but if I am to remain even somewhat optimistic, I will have to focus on the things I have accomplished. My inventory list grows slowly.

I have survived three blood clots in the last count, an operation after I thankfully "lined up," which allowed me to feel pain in its extreme. I've had five therapy sessions, which were done in my bed, and it left me with an idea of where I am destined to be slotted in the big evil universe. So much for the positive. Good air in, bad air out. As for the negative, well, it seems I will be a bit player on the big stage, a benchwarmer sitting in the dugout, a watcher, not a doer. That about covers the negative.

It is a grim reality, and it hit home only a week ago, by my reckoning, sometime during my first real therapy session. That is when denial left the building. Anger was meant to take its place, but it is a no-show for now. My anger is useless and self-indulgent, and although bargaining is supposed to come next, I fear I have skipped straight to depression.

The Heparin drip is gone, and my vertebrae had queued up like good little Englishman on a battlefield, straight and stoic. They have rebuilt and retooled my spinal column with bone paste from my hip, four small screws—never to be removed—and a straight piece of stainless steel (that appears about three inches long in the X-ray), which reconnects my spinal column from the fourth cervical vertebrae to the sixth. So after all that time in the "Frankenstein Monster" headgear, I was sure feeling better without it; the screws and the Halo attached to my head were gone. The tugging sensation that tried to detach my head from the rest of my body is gone, and two weeks later, I am now sporting a "whiplash" neck brace right out of central casting like I'm looking for a pending lawsuit. I was unceremoniously dropped into my first ever honest-to-goodness wheelchair by two nurses, and I fully intended to go down seven floors and begin my rehabilitation at that very moment. Still, the prolonged period on my back had left me weak and not a little nauseous. I came in at two hundred and six pounds, and I was now a poster boy for before and after weight loss. The after had me hovering between one fifty and one-fifty-five.

I blacked out the first four times they put me in the chair, and little stars were flying around my head for three full hours after they put me back into bed. It was a slow process.

Finally, they decided to put me in a girdle. Not a girdle exactly, but a truss of some kind that goes around my waist and gets pulled tight and then fastened with Velcro. It could be called a "corset;" it acts as a restraint to keep my guts and soft organs from sloshing around. It also acts as my stomach muscles, which used to do the job quite adequately, but they are no longer working, much like a good portion of the entire rest of my body. From the moment I put on the girdle, I progressed to the chair in tiny increments, much to the amusement of Wes, and after two days of false starts I arrived down in the "pit" for my introduction to therapy 101.

The pit is a large area designated for physical therapy. A mixture of Quadriplegics, Paraplegics, stroke victims, broken bones, and the brain-injured are all grouped in a large open room. Some perform little tricks like sitting, rolling over, and transferring, and others learn the big tricks, like bouncing balls against the wall and learning how to walk again.

The first time I was pushed there, I watched and observed as the circus rituals unfolded. It was my single worst day in the hospital, and perhaps my entire life. Finally, I believed I could see the future, and it scared the hell out of me. And there was Wes, who gave me the nod.

Wes was lifting minuscule fifteen-pound weakling weights over his head with a grimace of pain for every repetition in the free weight section. On the other hand, a considerably well-built individual and Paraplegic, Vince, did the same thing with substantially more weight and less grimace. At the same time, one brain-injured guy (who wasn't Thomas), driven by no-nonsense therapists, strived to put one foot in front of the other in an attempt to walk while holding precariously onto long horizontal bars. Vince gave me a big thumbs up and a wink, the latter sentiment being the only one I was capable of returning.

There were four king-size beds lined up against one wall and three more on the adjoining wall. They were covered with blue vinyl fitness mats, presumably making it easier to skid around. These mats were where the Quads hung out.

There were four Quads, including me, either a C5, a C6, or better. This is a popular spot to break your neck, close to where the cervical vertebrae meet the thoracic vertebrae. It is the weakest link. If I broke the damn thing at C7, there would be a good chance I'd get some hand movement and some triceps usage. "Them's the breaks," as Wes was so fond of saying.

The rest of the cast included Young Dean, who was seventeen and maybe a couple of weeks ahead of me, progress-wise. There were other fellow Quadriplegics. Scott, who looked about the same age, was nearing the end of his six-month stay, and there was another, Carl, who was about forty and had arrived three months ago. He looked surly and unapproachable. He was the final member of our four-man Quad relay team. On the first impression, neither one seemed very spry.

Scott was practicing his transfers from mat to chair and back to the mat again, and I couldn't help but think that he hadn't achieved much for a guy who had been here almost six months. Carl was trying to sit on the side of the bed all by himself. He had both arms out for balance, looking for all the world like he was 400 feet above the Earth, sitting there with a very small flagpole up his ass. Then there was Young Dean, who was just lying there looking pissed off.

Scott waved, welcoming the "new Quad on the block." Carl nodded a curt greeting—almost falling off his flag post—while Young Dean steadfastly ignored me and continued to look pissed off at the world. I assumed this was just a therapeutic step that I would have to endure when my time came to begin therapy. I could only aspire to look that pissed off until then. Now I was content to be overwhelmed and, admittedly, somewhat depressed.

Wes took time out to introduce me all around, and it was almost as if they knew me. I learned later that Wes had been getting a lot of mileage out of my imminent arrival, right to my current state of affairs. Their entire existence revolved around therapy and the seventh floor. The rest of the world had ceased to hold their interest. Nothing moved outside the hospital walls for these four to five people who were the current crop of the spinal cord injured. I was accepted into the club due to my injury. I spent the next two hours down in the pit that day, crying and dying inside while saying all the right things by rote. They were my brethren, my peer group. I was one of them, but I hated them. I was never more aware of how helpless I had become.

That day, the party finally broke up when Thomas T. Thomas, screaming obscenities, picked up his sturdy wooden cane and started swinging it over his head. At the same time, he desperately tried to push his wheelchair with his foot in the general direction of Wes. The therapists slowly and methodically evacuated the pit during his tirade, and I was never happier to be away from a place.

Bob has yet to die, but I hadn't seen Thomas for the better part of two weeks. It was sad to see he hadn't improved much since they had moved him out of our room. But of course, they moved him out right after "the incident." The fucking incident. The incident occurred because Thomas had continued his nighttime rants unabated until Wes finally snapped and tried to make good on his threat to suffocate him.

It was late one night; about that time everything shut down, and even most of the nurses were taking a catnap. I know I was sleeping—drugged-out peacefully—when Thomas started screaming. Loud whoops and wails made you imagine a procession of ambulances being chased by Hollywood-inspired wild Natives passing through our little hospital room. A hibernating bear couldn't have slept through the wailing. Wes was no exception, and he'd had enough.

Without a word or a sound, he pulled his wheelchair next to his bed and diligently transferred himself into it. I watched as he armed himself with a fluffy white pillow and stealthily wheeled himself over to Thomas's bed, and I knew it was for the sole intention of shutting him up for good. I should have said something then, I should have pulled the cord, but for some reason I kept quiet. Maybe I had finally had my fill of Thomas's late-night episodes as well. I like to think I kept quiet because I didn't know if Wes would follow through with his plan. But of course, anything I might have said wouldn't have made a lick of difference in any case, and I watched, fascinated, as Wes slowly and silently pushed himself toward Thomas.

During the incident, Bob's kettle started boiling more urgently. Maybe Bob was fucking aware. Who knows. It freaks me out thinking about it. I had applied the "vegetable" label on him from day one, but it seemed I wasn't going to be the only witness.

Thomas had been getting movement back in his arms, and along with the incessant caterwauling, he had taken to beating his arms against the bed rails. He had bruised himself mercilessly, and they were forced to pad the rails and put a new cast on his right wrist where he had chipped a bone, but the strength in his arms was all too apparent. Wes should have paid more attention.

The rail went down with a metallic clang that reverberated across the room. Wes had achieved step one of wheeling himself over to Thomas's bed, and step two was the rail. Then, on to step three, the pillow went over Thomas T. Thomas's face . . . but it was almost as if he had expected it, like he was playing possum. As soon as Wes put the pillow over his face, Thomas T. Thomas went fucking ballistic.

His entire body lurched sideways, and his arms stretched out and went around Wes's neck like he had been practicing for this very moment all along. They both ended up down in a heap. Wes screamed in surprise, and his wheelchair tipped over into his side of the room and upturned his bedside table. It crashed over on top of a biting, spitting, yelling Thomas, who had fallen out of his bed—leg cast, arm cast, and all—and now had his teeth firmly locked onto Wes's shoulder.

Wes's bedpan and his water jug, the stainless steel one Wes was so proud of because he wouldn't drink out of a "plastic water jug," had spilled over both of them, and there was a tangle of limbs and plaster and pieces of Wes's poorly built wheelchair.

"Pull the ripcord," Wes yelled over and over. "Pull the fucking ripcord."

I still couldn't reach it without a maximum effort at that time unless I reached way over my head, and now, when I look back, I'm not so sure I would have pulled it anyway.

In the ensuing melee, Wes had managed to grab his empty stainless steel water jug, and he was beating Thomas around the head with it. It made a dull clunking sound when it connected. Not to be outdone, Thomas maintained his bulldog-like bite on Wes's shoulder, and he was swinging his plaster-casted right arm around at anything unlucky enough to come within range. Neither one gave an inch. You could hear the metallic sound of the bedpan and the wheelchair pieces.

Thomas was still chewing on Wes's shoulder and flailing away with his cast, smashing at anything and everything. Wes was still hitting him in the head with the water jug until the nurses finally arrived to pull them apart. Wes's wheelchair was in pieces, and his tray table and Thomas's plaster cast were all in remnants, but the battle was still raging. Blood was everywhere, mixing with the spilled water and the plaster cast pieces. Both were screaming at the top of their lungs, Thomas whooping like a madman and Wes cursing and yelling just as loud. Finally, tiring out, they were both swinging for the knockout.

It has been referred to as "the incident" ever since. It took three nurses to pull them apart, calm them down, and get them back to bed. Wes received eight stitches in his shoulder and a tetanus shot. Thomas got a new cast and innumerable stitches in his head. So it was little wonder that Wes was the first one evacuated out of the pit when Thomas started swinging his sturdy wooden cane that day. Unfortunately, Thomas's sole mission in life since Wes's failed attempt to smother him was to kill Wes; and being inordinately stubborn and possessing a newfound survival instinct he never knew he had, Wes wasn't about to go quietly. Despite the eight stitches and the tetanus shot he'd received, he still tormented Thomas from afar every chance he got.

After "the incident," Thomas was subsequently moved to a private room in front of the nurse's station with a door that could be locked on the bottom or the top or both, should Thomas become inconsolable. Thomas was not about to escape at any rate, and though he had calmed down considerably since the first day I had met him, they still locked the bottom portion of the door and only kept the top part open. It was like the barn doors used at a farm when they were trying to keep the livestock safely tucked away without depriving them of fresh air and a glimpse of the outside. In retrospect, the nurses locked the bottom door to keep Wes out more so than to keep Thomas in.

When the nurses were busy and absent from the command center, which wasn't often, Wes would roll up to Thomas's room and pitch stuff at him over the bottom part of the door. Wadded up newspaper, rolls of tape, and cans of pop—full and empty—while calling him every demeaning word he could think up. If Thomas were to ever walk on his own, there was little doubt in my mind that he would pay a call on Wes and smother the living shit out of him.

Anyway, after the first interrupted-and-time-shortened non-therapy day at the pit, I somehow knew in my soul that I was not going to get better, and looking at the current crop of Quads was not unlike gazing into a crystal ball. Denial had passed me by, and it was replaced by depression. It was a lassitude and a torpor more befitting a defeated, hopeless individual waiting to die as painlessly as possible than a thirty-year-old man with the rest of his life stretched out ahead of him. Depression is an unrelenting bitch.

CHAPTER EIGHTEEN

DEPRESSION STILL

BOB HAS BEEN REPLACED. HIS name is Mr. Mawani, Althuna has informed me, and he suffers from something that sounds suspiciously like Green Beret disease. It paralyzes you entirely from the neck down, but strangely enough, you can fully recover on the whim of this odd disease, or the downside, you could remain forever in stasis, hoping for a reprieve. It intrigues me. I make a mental note to find out more about this disease. Since my stay here, I have become a back-seat doctor. I spend hours poring over medical texts that would not have even slightly piqued my interest a month ago. It all started when I began reading articles and books about spinal cord injuries in the hospital library (everything I never wanted to know); I soon progressed to other debilitating diseases from there. I was lost and trapped, and information was my friend.

Bob's replacement, Mr. Mawani—a tall man of East Indian descent— would be considered ancient on the senior lawn bowling circuit. His skin is parchment-thin, and his face is sunken and drawn, emphasizing his large, hooked nose. He pretty much looks mummified, and he is feeble with a collection of angles and bones that might weigh in at about ninety pounds, but his body belies his voice, which is anything but frail and delicate.

The day he showed up, his entrance was preceded by a seemingly endless parade of East Indian women and children dressed in wild-colored flowing robes, and they gathered around his bed like royal attendants. At the same time, he barked orders with the cadence of a drill sergeant. I don't have the foggiest notion of what he is saying because I don't speak Hindi or whatever language he's speaking, but the message is unmistakable. He expects total compliance. They put cold cloths on his forehead, feed him, hold the water jug up so he can drink from the straw, and tuck the blankets around him, almost as if their very existence depended on his immediate comforts. They stumble over each other to do his bidding. The cynical side of me immediately wonders just how much money this old withered, parsimonious, skeleton-man with the chainsaw voice has stashed away, because I'm betting everyone is lining up for their slice of the inheritance pie.

I am a mute witness to these proceedings because nobody had the foresight to pull the privacy curtain, which stays open all day with the steady stream of people coming and going. I was given a rain check from therapy that morning due to a higher-than-average temperature and the confusion caused by the death of Bob and his new replacement. I had been planning a relaxing morning free from distraction. At least that was my intention until this shrunken older man was ushered in and started abusing everyone around him in a strange tongue. I am now wishing I could pull the ripcord, and for once, the sight of Wes returning from his morning therapy buoys me instead of annoys me.

"Who's the rug rider, Wagner?" is the first thing he says as he rolls up to my bed after passing in front of the jam-packed area where Mr. Mawani is casting aspersions on his immediate family. He has switched to English now, and I sense it is for the benefit of both Wes and myself. His accent is thick, and I believe he has just called one of the older males a dung eater (or an "eater" of something equally unpleasant). He wants us to know he has this situation well in hand, and all his ducks are in a row. I suspect he is trying to either make a good impression on us or intimidate us, although I can't figure out why he would feel compelled to do either for the life of me.

As soon as he switches languages, the two oldest and gaudily garbed East Indian women start keening and moaning as if the steady spate of aspersions carries more weight when spoken in English, and they bow their heads.

"His name's Mr. Mawani," I tell Wes above the barking of the prone Mr. Mawani and the lament of the two older women.

"What's his story?" asks Wes, screwing up his face in disgust. Loud noises adversely affect Wes, and it's beginning to sound like an outdoor bazaar in downtown New Delhi in the small hospital room.

"He's got something called Green Beret disease," I inform him loudly.

"Sounds to me like he's got fucking Loudmouth disease, or he's just downright hard of hearing," says Wes, and with that said, he yells at the top of his lungs, "SHUT THE FUCK UP, YOU RAG HEAD BASTARDS."

It has the desired effect. The whole pack falls silent and turns and stares at Wes in disbelief. Prejudice is one thing. Out and out disrespect is another. I'm staring at Wes, too, because I feel somewhat responsible for some inexplicable reason.

"What's your problem?" he says while surreptitiously wheeling himself over to the other side of the room towards his bed. Since "the incident," Wes is now situated in the space directly across from mine. He is against the window, where Thomas used to be, so I know he's going for the racquet.

Wes has acquired a tennis racquet since his failed attempt at a good old-fashioned smothering. I shouldn't say he "acquired" one because he always had it, but it was put away in a locker behind his bed with his other personal stuff. He now carries it with him whenever he can, everywhere but therapy. He tells everyone he needs it for protection because he is allergic to bee stings, which is an almost valid excuse. After all, the bees fly into the unscreened open windows on the seventh floor like they own the place, as if there's some secret flower stash that only they know about. Of course, they just as quickly fly out again, but the unfortunate ones that do get confused and trapped get forehanded and backhanded by Wes, who, by his account, was a great tennis player in his walking days. However, I know (and everyone else suspects) that Wes carries the tennis racquet because Thomas T. Thomas is never far away. Still, I let him get away with the bee excuse because he does seem to enjoy whacking around bees. Hospital life is ninety percent boredom at best anyway. Wes eschews reading like it's a harrowing experience to avoid at all costs, so if spiking hapless bees against the wall keeps him busy, then so much the better. At least *I* can get some reading done. Meanwhile, the Mawanis continue to stare at Wes as he inches closer to his bed and his prized racquet, but their response is not quite what either of us expects.

"So sorry," Mr. Mawani says. "Oh, so very, very sorry." I try not to laugh at his pronunciation of "very," as it comes out sounding more like "belly-belly" than "very-very." "My family is just upset, so belly upset," he continues, and his family bows their heads in unison as if to put an exclamation point on Mr. Mawani's apology. It's now our turn to stare, but Wes has regained his tennis racquet, confidence, and brash attitude.

"Don't let it happen again," he says, and he *boings* the racquet strings up against the palm of his other hand for effect. It's laughable watching the Mawanis react to this implied threat, if that's what it could be called. They cringe with every *boing*. It's like watching school kids shrink while the teacher whacks a ruler in their open palm. Wes has just achieved bully status.

Mr. Mawani snaps off a couple more orders, and his family all bustle out as one. But before they go, they nod or bow in Wes's direction like he is some evil yet possibly benevolent god, and he must be appeased to keep their father or husband alive and happy.

"I am so belly pleased to meet you, and my name is Mr. Mawani. Unfortunately, I am having some belly bad pains and paralysis right now, so I cannot shake your hand as is da custom. Please, forgive me."

"You're forgiven," I tell him. "My name is Wagner, and this is Wes," who is still unconsciously racquet-smashing against his palm. It is fucking annoying.

"You are being belly good at tennis then, Mr. Wes?" he asks Wes, who seems to be a million miles away.

"Huh? Oh yeah, I am being 'belly-belly' good at tennis," he says absently, and then his face brightens up as if a great idea had just occurred to him. "You know," he starts, looking and sounding very serious, "I think you might want to be across the room beside me. That space is vacant, and it's right close to the bathroom. Way more privacy and way more convenient." He's right, of course, it is close to the bathroom, and I'm about to point out that Wes himself just gave up that very spot not so long ago, but I want to see where this is going.

"Besides," he continues, "Bob was the fellow that used to be in that spot, and he is barely cold and dead, and it's upsetting to see someone take his place so quickly. I also think it's bad luck to take the recently deceased's place. I can still smell death from that corner."

"What the hell . . ." I start, and Wes cuts me off immediately by slapping the head of his aluminum racquet on the frame of my bed. It sends shivers up the bed right into my shoulders and neck. It stops me from asking all the obvious questions. Since when did Wes give a flying fuck about anybody but himself?

"Think about it, Mawani, a guy just died there, a great guy, a friend to us all. It's hard to see you suddenly set up camp in his place. It's like sacrilegious or something." During Wes's little discourse, the whole time he's banging home his points by hitting the racquet on my bed frame, and I can't wait for him to finish. "Besides," he continues with another clang, "that corner is cursed. The guy before Bob, sleeping in that very spot, also died suddenly during the night. Nobody knows why."

For all I know, this might be true, but whether it is or not is immaterial. The die is cast. After much consideration, Mr. Mawani has decided to move. I think the part about that particular corner being cursed was the turning point. He has already asked Wes to summon the nurse, and Wes is only too happy to do this.

I've given up trying to figure out what the big deal is. I'm just glad Wes has stopped banging on my metal bed frame. When Althuna and Pam come in, they reluctantly agree to move Mr. Mawani—he's pretty insistent. I ask her to pull the privacy curtain around me, and I go down for a nap while Wes oversees the entire move. Another day is in the books, and I make a mental note to ask Wes why he wants to place Mr. Mawani in the space he used to occupy.

CHAPTER NINETEEN

MORE DEPRESSION,
I CAN'T SHAKE IT

THE DAYS GO BY, AND day forty is quickly upon us. Mr. Mawani fits right in. He is polite to a point, well-mannered, and he is filled with exciting stories about West Africa, where he had a tiny carpet and furniture store. Unfortunately, he sold out and decided to pursue his ambitions in Canada after a falling out with his second wife's family, who were politically connected and disapproved of the marriage. He is currently on his third wife, and he is doing quite well in the export-import carpet business. He has three outlets in Calgary alone. By all accounts, Mr. Mawani is stinking rich, owns many properties in India, and his children from his many marriages never fail to visit. Their visits are also a bonus for Wes and me.

Mr. Mawani's children bring him armloads of treats and homemade dishes that taste as delectable as they smell. He accepts these offerings with the grace of Buddha, thanking them profusely, but he takes great pains to explain to them that they are not deserving of any of his money. This only spurs them to more extraordinary acts of loyalty. Mr. Mawani is pampered, primped, handfed beyond reasonable expectations, and receives enough food to feed half the seventh floor.

Wes and I, and sometimes my wife, enjoy these little authentic tastes of Indian cuisine. Curries and chutneys with lamb and chicken, pickled vegetables, basmati rice, and curried whole baby potatoes with spicy pearl onions are far superior to the mundane hospital food they placate us with—and infinitely more nutritious. Yes, life on the seventh floor would not be all-bad if only I weren't still basically paralyzed from the shoulders down. That thought never leaves my mind.

Therapy helps. Although I'm not very proficient, I get better as I learn to "work with what I have." That is the mantra they are drilling into my head, and I'm not alone. Scott, Carl, and Young Dean get the same pep talks. Wes gets only minimum encouragement, and Vince the almost upright Para is right there with the therapists, cheering our accomplishments, as meager as they might be. Unfortunately, good therapists are a cross between prison guards and dog trainers; they threaten and cajole with equal amounts of enthusiasm, and the rewards are slim pickings.

I can almost lift my right arm to shoulder level if I lean back real far, and I can now stay in the wheelchair for four to five hours in one go. Any more, and the bedsore monsters will come up and grab me by the ass, and when they bite they never let go. So, bedsores are now a fundamental part of my sad little life, as I have learned from *Doctor Doom* himself.

He comes by semi-daily, and on one of his visits he brought along a video. Vince the almost upright Para, Wes, Scott, Carl, Young Dean, and I were forced to watch it, and I can't speak for them, but it scared the Billy B. Jesus out of me. It was a lot like one of those "worst-case scenario" drunk driving seminars where they show you mangled corpses for shock value, hoping it'll be enough to deter you from drinking and driving. In this case, they offer you ulcerous, suppurating flesh and the inevitable onset of sepsis, gangrene, and all manners of afflictions that befall the lazy Quads or Paras if they don't shift their butt, feet, and legs to achieve maximum blood flow. I darn near puked looking at the desecrated and ruined skin oozing yellow and green gunk.

My wife also watched the video, and she was equally appalled. In mid-sentence now, she often gets behind me and lifts my ass off the seat cushion because I can't do that myself as of yet. She massages my feet, even though

I can't feel them, and she constantly reminds me to stay in the wheelchair only for abbreviated periods. All in all, she has been very supportive.

But my wife has never faltered in her belief that I will improve and fully recover. She clings to that three-month deadline like a drowning ship-wrecked sailor hanging onto a life preserver in the middle of a cold, unfriendly sea while sharks of doubt circle incessantly. She pretends not to see the sharks. Her emotional and physical well-being depends on it. I rue the day when the sharks break through her carefully constructed barricades and rip her to shreds.

My wife is essentially an outwardly strong person, always in control, stoic in defeat, and gracious in victory. Well, maybe a tad selfish, but not so you'd notice. She doesn't take her perfect pill every morning, but who does? Still, her sense of humor rarely deserts her, which is one of the things I love about her. However, she expects a lot from people. She can be very patient, especially when she has to explain something or train someone for a position in any restaurant and, more importantly, the one we will soon possess. She can forgive almost anything; the keyword here, though, is "almost." If I remain a Quad, she will never forgive me. I know this to be true as well as I know my name.

She relies on me for support. Our relationship was built on this premise. I'm the leaning post, the free parking space on the giant Monopoly board, and her compass all rolled into one. Together we can take on the big, imperfect, ugly, old world. Alone we're unfinished, unrefined, and undone. The restaurant enterprise will suffer accordingly. I must improve or downright heal, or we're drowning together. In the meantime, she visits almost every day, hiding her disappointment and offering unflagging encouragement when I need it. She took a job at the same Keg that we had left to travel back to Lethbridge on that fateful night. That same night that I have relived a million times and no doubt will never stop reliving. Mark hired her, the same Mark whose car I so callously dented with a golf ball in the parking lot. I'm not sure whether she was hired because Mark felt sorry for her or because she is a darn good waitress. Quite frankly, I don't care, and we certainly do need the money, so I am glad she got hired, and I'm not about to look a gift horse in the mouth. Restaurants under construction, such as ours, generate zero income.

My wife has also taken great pains to visit during therapy sessions. She has learned to transfer me, and she has a general idea of what to expect during bowel management days. That's what they euphemistically call it, while it is as simple as sticking a suppository up your ass and sitting you on a commode chair over a toilet.

It's brutally undignified, and since all Quads and Paras have bowel management days simultaneously, Young Dean, Scott, Wes, Vince the upright Para, and I are forced to sit over a row of toilets like crows perched on a wire with only a half-wall of melamine separating us. Carl is an absentee. He must be on a different schedule, or he flatly refuses to shit, which would not surprise me. We try to make this more bearable by making the requisite bawdy toilet jokes and emitting grotesque sounds for no apparent reason other than we are embarrassed to be there in the first place. I used to go to great lengths to ensure the bathroom door stayed locked when I was young while taking a bathroom break. At times, I even propped chairs in front of the door should my siblings find sufficient reason to pick the lock. Now it seems that my bowel management days are public domain. I believe that dignity must be suspended and eventually buried if I hope to get on with my new life. My wife will have to be a part of this. Time will tell.

There are always new developments as the days pass, though. I remember when Wes's fiancée came to visit him. I had no inkling that he had any significant other, let alone a fiancée. He never mentioned a relationship of any kind until she inexplicably showed up one afternoon. She introduced herself through tear-filled eyes and did little more than cry when she talked to Wes. He pulled the oxymoronic *privacy curtain* around them minutes after she arrived, but I heard their conversation as plain as day, as if I was right in there with them.

"So stop crying," said Wes.

"I can't help it," said his fiancée. "We planned to buy a house, have a large family, love each other forever."

"Yeah, I know all about the 'sickness and in health' bullshit, and if you can hang on another couple of months, we can still have all of those things."

The tears stopped then. "I can't," she says. "I want a normal life." Her voice carried a hard edge at that point. It was a complete turnaround, and I didn't need to see her face to know that she had given this a lot of thought and had come to her decision long before entering the hospital room. I could feel Wes die by degrees behind the privacy curtain. He never begged or pleaded, to his credit; he never said anything, not a peep, but his silence spoke volumes. I imagined him behind the curtain, turning his head away and dismissing her. The silence seemed to stretch out forever, but it was probably only a couple of minutes until she felt the need to speak again.

"So that's it then," she started, "that's the end? You're not going to say anything?" The silence continued. Stubborn silence was Wes's only response. It was the first time in the short stretch I had known him that he was at a loss for words. His fiancée had sucked the entire life force out of him.

"I'll pack up your clothes then and take them over to your parents' place," she continued. "We'll split the trailer, and I'll pay you out after selling it. Are you sure there's nothing you want to say? Nothing at all?" But Wes, the misery vampire, remained quiet, and I thought it best to do the same, although I was chomping at the bit to get a couple of digs in. Wes's fiancée was not endearing herself to me, not by a long shot. If Wes didn't have the guts to call her a self-serving bitch, maybe I should do it for him.

I never got that opportunity though. She started crying again, and she left in a hurry holding a Kleenex over her face without a word of goodbye. Wes acted like she had never visited, and I never mentioned her visit. Some things are just better left alone.

CHAPTER TWENTY

EVEN MORE DEPRESSION, BUT MOSTLY ANGER WITH A SMALL BIT OF BARGAINING

IT'S LIKE BEING IN PRISON. You find yourself mentally checking off days on the calendar. It is day forty-six, forty-six stinking rotten lousy days since I quit being Randy Wagner the walking guy. I am now "Wag the Quad," more or less the name Wes bestowed on me on our first meeting. My wife hates my new name, but I find it necessary.

"How can you just give up?" she asks me.

"I haven't given up as much as I've given in," I tell her. "I can't be both guys at once because then therapy would be a waste of time, and believe me when I say that I would be in here forever if I waited all humble and submissive while someone produced a cure-all magic pill. So, thinking that perhaps this may be all the feeling I get back makes me try harder."

"Don't talk like that. Look at what's returned already." She has a point there, as I can now lift my arms almost up to my shoulders. That is until my triceps refuse to work, and then my arms slam back to the top of my head as gravity kicks in, but this is not big news. *Doctor Doom* told me that my triceps would be useless because, at the point where I broke my vertebrae and separated my spinal cord, this is considered normal. I could reasonably expect to get the feeling back in my thumb, some shoulder movement, and almost complete biceps contraction. The top of my forearm would have some sensation but not much strength, and I would be able to raise my wrist backward but not on the palm side. The inside of my arm would be without feeling or muscle tone, and I would never arm wrestle again—okay, he didn't say that last part. So far, *Doctor Doom* was right on all counts. I had seen the X-rays more than once, and I had truly *separated* my cervical vertebrae between C5 and C6. There was a mess of bone fragments floating around before my operation that stabilized my spinal cord.

"What's returned is what I expected, nothing more," I inform my wife for what seems like the trillionth time.

"Doctor Dumars also said that as time went on, some 'sparing' might occur, which means you could reasonably expect to get your hands back and some feeling in your legs."

"Sparing is for partial separation. Mine is complete. I have to face the facts. Did you not see the X-rays?"

"You're not trying hard enough," my wife says, and for the first time since I have known her, I wish to hurt her. I have the urge to smash her in the face.

I am not a happy Quad on day forty-six. I am not in the mood for "maybes" and "what-ifs," and I'm certainly not in the mood to hear how I'm not trying hard enough, but I choke on my reply and try to understand where she is coming from. Unfortunately, some people—and it appears my wife is lumped into the "some people" category—don't seem to grasp that no amount of effort will make you walk again, or even make one lousy finger move for that matter. The current is cut, and there is no power. You can't *will* the connection. That particular bulb is burned out. You can flick the switch until it snows in Mexico, but you will only be able to move those body parts that come under the direct control of the synapses that are still firing.

What I can do is improve my strength. I can adapt and use other muscles for a movement it wasn't originally meant to make, and I can compensate by using my imagination. But try as I might, I cannot, by sheer force of will, cajole, coax, threaten, or otherwise persuade or induce movement out of a body part, any body part, below the injury site where I have irreparably damaged my spinal cord.

I remember on a television show I watched one time—I think it was an *Ironside* rerun—when the hero, who happened to be wheelchair-bound, had only minutes to save a small girl trapped in the path of a runaway bus or train or some such thing. Through concentration and what looked like nothing short of mind power alone, Ironside was able to revive his legs and stagger the two or three steps necessary to push the small girl to safety. Well, I now know that it was pure Hollywood crap. In real life, the hero can't get out of his chair unless he levitates, which is just about as likely as his legs suddenly working, and the small girl in real life is just so much as roadkill. I hate real life, but it's where I have to live.

My wife will realize this soon enough because I can't try any harder, and it's taking all my available willpower to stay positive as it is. Further conversation is suspended, however, by the appearance of a large young man with two canes who looks intent on talking to me. He adeptly walks into the room with his arm canes (like Vince the upright Para would eventually do). He nods in my direction, slides a chair over, and sits down with a big sigh. It is a chair usually occupied by one of Mr. Mawani's many immediate family members, but Mr. Mawani is down in therapy at the moment. With a wave of his hand and a quick nod, he indicates that my wife and I should finish our talk regardless of his presence, which my wife and I have no intention of doing. I am still a private person and have absolutely no desire to air my laundry in public. He waits patiently, though, and stares intently at his fingernails while trying unsuccessfully to remain unobtrusive. He moves his canes around briefly, but he is in no hurry to get on with the rest of his life.

"Can I help you there, partner?" I ask him. He looks strangely familiar. I think I've seen him skulking around before this, but he's one of those unassuming sorts that you forget about minutes after passing him in the hall.

"Well, I came to talk to Randy Wagner, and if that's who you are, then I'm in the right place. But please, don't let me interrupt."

"A little late for that, don't you think?" I say, still stinging from the accusation that I am not trying hard enough. I'm not in the mood for strange visitors, regardless of their motives.

"I'm here from Social Assistance," he says.

"In what regard? If you're peddling religion, you can hobble right back out the door and take it somewhere else, Cane-Boy." I felt terrible about the Cane-Boy comment immediately after I said it, but I let it lie.

"Nope, not religion. Counseling."

"Oh good, he could use someone to talk to," says my wife before I can tell him that I have about the same respect for counseling as I do for organized religion.

"I can?" I say, closing one eye and looking at her sideways.

"You can," she assures me. "I'll leave you two to talk. I have to go to work anyway. Maybe talking about your injury might give you a different perspective."

"I do talk. I talk to Wes, Scott, Carl, Vince the upright Para, and Young Dean if I have to."

"I meant talking to someone who isn't morbid or cynical. Those guys all have a dim view of the future."

I couldn't argue there. Most of our conversations were pretty skewed because of our new viewpoint, as we were all sentenced to the rest of our lives in a wheelchair with no chance for parole or time off for good behavior, except maybe Vince the upright Para. This new guy may have walked in with a couple of canes, but he had still walked in nonetheless (the lucky bastard), so his perspective differed. It had to. So, to me, that meant he had nothing new to offer, and I had no desire to talk to him. I had to count myself among the people on the seventh floor who had "a dim view of the future." My wife is adamant, though, and she gives me a look that conveys her opinion of my opinion.

"Okay," I say, kissing my wife goodbye as she goes off to work. I've decided to see what the new guy might have to offer me in the way of perspective. What did I have to lose? On the eighth-floor roof, Wes was smoking a joint with Scott, Mr. Mawani was still down in therapy, and I had an hour to kill before dinner arrived.

"So, what's your story?" I ask the new guy, in a hurry to get to the point. Since my injury, I've been impatient with people in general and walking people in particular. I can spend an hour trying to put a quarter in the Coke machine or thirty minutes trying to dial a number on the telephone, but I can't abide walking people who won't get to the point. I shouldn't say I am impatient with all walking people, primarily those who are just offering advice.

Vince the upright Para is an exception to this rule.

Sorry, Vince the *almost* upright Para. He was in a motorcycle accident, and they never expected him to live. However, he surprised everyone, and he regained his consciousness and strength, which says a lot because he could probably bench-press a truck before the accident. With the use of two canes that attach to his forearms, and with the help of this exoskeleton-like device that keeps his legs straight—though it looks like it came off the set of a science fiction movie—Vince can move forward slowly but painfully in the upright position. For Vince, this is a monumental achievement in itself, not only because he weighs in the neighborhood of two hundred fifty pounds, has tattoos, earrings, and brass knuckles in the guise of rings included, but also because he has a steel rod that keeps his spine lined up. The pain involved in moving at all is supposed to be near unbearable. All this, and Vince the almost upright Para never stops smiling and joking. We do give him a ribbing in turn, but this guy in front of me isn't Vince the upright Para, but I'll still give him the time of day if he can spark my interest. He does make me think to myself that maybe Vince will be in the same boat one day. This guy looks soft, and Vince the almost upright Para is a rock. Hell, if anyone is walking out of here, it's Vince.

"I'm a counselor," he starts.

"You said that already. So what makes you uniquely qualified to counsel the likes of me? And don't tell me it's because you have some distant relative who sits in a wheelchair, died of cancer, or some such bullshit."

"Ah, so you've noticed that every walking person has a sad story to tell you about a loved one or a family member that's sharing your bad fortune. Good, that's good, but you know they just do that to get closer so they can relate a little to your condition. It makes them feel like they're on your level, like they know where you're coming from."

"And you're not going to do that?"

"I am. You see, I was a C3 Quad about four years ago, but I got a lot of 'sparing.' It was a partial separation, not quite in your league, but I do remember what it was like to lay in bed and think that I would never walk again, so I can at least share with you on that level."

"What's your name?" I ask him. Despite my initial misgivings, his story is better than most, and he has an easy way about him. He's quick to smile and his four years of experience trumps my forty-six days by a country mile. I notice the little worm-like ridge of scar tissue on his throat just above his collar. "Hey, is that a tracheotomy scar?" I ask him.

"You bet. I stopped breathing on the scene. I think the first responders used a jackknife and a drinking straw. They made a right mess of it, but it kept me alive. Name's Charlie, by the way."

"How long were you in?"

"Nine months. I had some problems with bedsores. I figured I would lie in bed until medical science made a breakthrough. Everything seemed pointless."

"How long in the Halo?"

"One month."

"Let me guess. You fell out of a fucking pickup truck?"

"Nope, I took a wrong turn skiing."

"Okay, so what can you do for me?" He'd passed the test. We had established common ground like a couple of Vietnam vets or ex-cons with prison tattoos on their knuckles that did a stretch in the same prison.

"I can listen. I'm here for you. Maybe I could give you some advice that might help you get set up with the right people when you get out and get back on your feet, so to speak." He laughs at his joke and then immediately switches tracks. "Was that your wife that just left?"

"Yep."

"Are you close?"

"I did marry her. We're inseparable."

"No such thing."

"That's where you're dead wrong, buddy, and if you mention my wife again, you'll go on my list."

"Your list?"

"Yeah, my list. It's a list I'm making in my head of the people who piss me off while I'm in my wheelchair. It's the list of people I plan to wind up and kick in the nuts really fucking hard. I plan to do this later when I walk again, and I've got an excellent memory."

"Well, I wouldn't want to get on your list. How many people are on it already?"

"Three and counting; well, four cause Wes is on it twice, so you can see how easy it would be to bump you to the head of the list, so don't piss me off."

"I'll try not to. What's your story anyway? I hear you crashed a car, did a Humpty Dumpty on your noggin, took twenty or thirty stitches."

"Yep, only I think it was more like sixteen or seventeen," and somewhere deep down, weirdly, I feel almost proud of my stitches. They are battle scars; they are like little badges of honor. These thoughts are way too strange for me. I have to get back to safer ground.

"How do you get to be a counselor?" I ask him.

"You ask. It's a volunteer thing."

"You ask to talk to people like me?"

"Yeah, glutton for punishment, that's me. But maybe I feel guilty because I got to walk again, and most C3s don't. Maybe it's because only someone who went through the same thing that you're going through now can understand where your head is at, and that's me. So I guess I'm attracted to kindred souls."

"So, no religion."

"Yeah, I heard you're not very tolerant of preachers or priests," he points out.

"You got that right. That priest in the church downstairs is on my list, but how would you know that? Who have you been talking to?"

"I talked to Doctor Dumars, *Doctor Doom* as you call him. I also talked to Dean and Carl. Only Carl doesn't talk much. He won't even tell me how he got his injury. I talk to Scott, a good guy, a positive guy, who loses his way now and again, but Scott is on his way out. And when I can, I'll shoot the shit with Vince because he knows more jokes than anyone I've ever met. I used to talk to Wes too, but Wes is a lost cause. He has far too many issues for me. I hear his fiancée booked on him, and he went psycho and tried to smother a brain-injured guy."

"Yeah, something like that, but we don't talk about it. Young Dean brought it up once, and Wes belted him in the head with that aluminum racquet he packs around. You sure seem to know a lot of shit going on around here."

"Yeah, I hear you guys get together and have a meeting of sorts every morning in the lounge and drink the nurse's coffee. I can't blame you, though. That other freeze-dried shit they give you here tastes like it's strained through some old gym socks or day-old underwear. So, what's that game you got them all playing? The 'What Would You Rather Have' game or something like that."

"I call it the 'What's Better Sweepstakes'; get it right. It just came up one morning, and I guess it's become somewhat of a preoccupation."

"How do you play?" he asks with genuine interest.

"Well, you just come up with a scenario, a disease, or a condition, and you compare it to a similar or not-so-similar situation, and then you try to decide what's better. A simple example would be: what's better? Being blind or being deaf, or saying something less drastic, like losing your little finger instead of losing your little toe, that kind of thing."

"Kind of a grim-sounding game."

"Not really. It's just a perspective exercise. Kind of an extension on the old maxim, every Quad would be happy to be a Para, and every Para wants to walk."

"You'd be happy to be a Paraplegic?"

"Fucking-A right I would, Charlie. It would be a cakewalk compared to being a Quad."

"Neither one is a cakewalk."

"Granted, but that's not what the 'What's Better Sweepstakes' is all about."

"Give me another example."

"You know Thomas?"

"Yeah, that's the young guy Wes tried to shut up for good. The guy who refused to be smothered."

"Yep, that's the guy. So, now Thomas is a tard. Pardon the expression. Niceties don't fucking matter much to me anymore. He took a brain blow, and even though it's looking like he might walk again, he'll always be about as sharp as a watermelon. So, what's better? Being a Quad who can still think? Remember, reason and converse. Or being a tard who can walk and barely wipe his ass? Someone who doesn't remember what day it is and might spend his life staring at a blank TV screen thinking he's watching the Olympics when in reality he's watching a *Bugs Bunny* rerun?"

"Whoa, whoa, that's a lot of choices."

"No contest when you think about it. You spend a lifetime collecting memories. I wouldn't want those messed with, and they define you. Your memories are a vast collection of experiences and encounters that shape your life and make you who and what you are."

"So, conversely, Thomas has no quality of life?"

"Sure, if you want to boil it all down to that one catchphrase, then sure, Thomas has no quality of life, and maybe he has no reason to live, but he's still better off than some people. He can at least feel pleasure and pain, happiness and disappointment, and he can still emote and give love in some ways if that matters to him. He's somewhat aware, and that counts for something. It sounds corny to anyone else, but the quality of life is a pretty transient concept. That's what makes the 'What's Better Sweepstakes' such an interesting game."

"Young Dean, as you call him, told me about one of your scenarios."

"Bet I can guess which scenario. It goes something like this: What's better, being a seventeen-year-old virgin who became a Quad before he knew what he was missing, or becoming a Quad at thirty knowing precisely what you're missing?"

I do remember posing this one to Young Dean. It screwed up his day. Hell, it screwed up his week and his month. He insisted it was better not knowing what sex was all about, while Wes insisted, in his Wes-like way, that he'd rather have fucked "five fat chicks and a corpse" as opposed to never having had sex at all before his accident. I can't say I agreed with Wes entirely, but he was on the right track and of a like mind, give or take the corpse part. Young Dean threw his coffee cup at the sink that day as we delved further into the possibilities. It shattered into a hundred pieces. I think he secretly agreed with Wes, except (I'm hoping) not the corpse part. Even thinking about that makes me shudder.

"You can see how that might have upset Young Dean," says Charlie, interrupting my thoughts.

"So what?" I say right back. "Upsetting someone on the seventh floor doesn't bother me in the least. I have developed an 'every man for himself' type of attitude, and it's easier to get through the day without the requisite moral roadblocks."

"Young Dean's parents would like to know if you would talk to him?"

"Talk to Young Dean? Is that what this is all about? I always talk to Young Dean."

"It's not entirely about that, I'm still here for you if *you* want to talk, but I'm worried about Dean specifically."

"Worried about Young Dean, huh? Well then, you're a lot dumber than I thought. Young Dean is an attention-seeking little weasel who pulls everyone's chain until he gets a response."

"Do you know he tried to kill himself last night? He was up on the eighth-floor roof, and he was trying to throw himself off."

"Yeah, right, like that has a high success rate when you can't even lift your ass off the chair. The roof railing is four feet tall and topped with spikes. It just ain't going to happen, I checked. Oh, and last week Dean tried to hang himself with the ripcord that you pull to summon a nurse. I think he succeeded in falling out of bed and bruising his ribs and his ego. And I believe the week before that, he was sticking his head in the elevator doors as they were closing, which also has a low success ratio. If Young Dean really wanted to kill himself, he has this failsafe device that Wes and I designed."

"What are you talking about?"

"The toilet spear, or as Wes calls it, the plunger lance. It's a little clunky, but we'll worry about the name if we patent it."

"You've lost me, toilet spear? Plunger lance?" And as he's trying to picture this concept, Wes returns from sucking on a joint or two, if he and Scott are running true to form. Of course, Wes's eyes are red, but there are enough drugs around here to keep a truckload of junkies happy, so red eyes are not necessarily a dead giveaway to being stoned.

"Hey, if it isn't Chucklehead, the loser boy amateur counselor and all-around pain in the ass," says Wes. "Picking Wagner's brain, are you? You'll find out he's the sanest one in here except me. You're wasting your fucking precious time."

"Thanks, Wes," I say, wondering if that simple distinction merits a thank you, as Wes seems to be the least sane person on this floor, Thomas included.

"What's a toilet spear, Wes? Or a plunger lance, if you like?" asks Charlie, who will not deter. This question causes Wes to laugh for several minutes, lending credence to my suspicion that he's stoned out of his head. He can't stop laughing, but he's holding his hand up, so I know he wants to explain, and I wait while he composes himself. After all, I may have conceived it, but Wes built it with the tools at hand (give or take some duct tape I had smuggled in from the outside). Of course, since "the incident," Wes isn't allowed things like duct tape.

"No, really, Wes," says Charlie, not sharing the joke. "I'm curious. What the hell is a plunger lance or a toilet spear?"

"It's kind of a do-it-yourself suicide kit for Quads. I tried like hell to develop a catchier name, but it wasn't that big of a deal."

"What?" Charlie is beyond curious now and more than a little worried.

"Don't be so serious, Chucklehead," says Wes. "It's just a broomstick sharpened to a point on one end with a toilet plunger shoved in and duct-taped onto the other end, and there's a little holder I fashioned from a bent fork so anyone, even a useless Quad, can hold it out straight. We built it, especially for Young Dean. This way he can wind up his electric wheelchair to five miles an hour, hold the pointy part against his chest, run the plunger part against a brick wall and impale himself on the broomstick. Sort of like jousting, but the brick wall always wins. If he gets up enough speed and hits the wall just right, the sharpened end should stick right through him and come out the other side."

"You gave him this?" says Charlie, incredulous.

"Yeah, so what? Wagner thought it up. He's the idea guy."

"So what? So what. Dean is on edge. He's depressed, clinically depressed. You don't think that *maybe* he might use it?"

"That's the whole point," says Wes.

"No, it isn't," I insert myself. "The point is Young Dean will never use it."

"Not yet," says Charlie, "but that's not the point either."

"That is indeed the point," I state emphatically. "Young Dean is looking for everyone to feel sorry for him. He wants attention and will never use the stinking toilet spear. If he had been serious about killing himself, he would have used it by now. You don't plan on taking it away from him, do you?"

"Yes, I do."

"Wes worked a long time on that."

"So what?"

"So, so you're empowering Young Dean and belittling Wes. How do you think that makes Wes feel?" I'm trying to be facetious, but it goes over Charlie's head.

"I don't care," he states pretty firmly. He sounds somewhat pissed off, and this guy's a counselor? Apparently I'm not taking this seriously enough, but fuck him, he hasn't had to put up with Young Dean daily. One day we played the game, and I introduced the one *what if* that had been dogging me for weeks. "What if," I said, "you could kill somebody to regain the use of your limbs?" A dumb premise, but it creates a moral dilemma. Take a life to get yours back, a fair trade if you could pick a convicted felon. Too easy, so we took that off the board. It came down to murdering a complete stranger. Wes, of course, volunteered that he could strangle a dozen people to get walking again. Vince the upright Para said no, not under any circumstances. Carl looked around like there might be someone right there he could murder. Scott said maybe, which shows you just how fucked up Quads are because I shared his sentiment at the time. Young Dean just insisted that he would want to pick the person he killed.

"I'm just thinking of Dean," says Charlie, still sounding worried.

"I thought you were here for us. *All* of us. Me, Wes, Carl, Scott, and Vince the upright Para," I said sarcastically.

"I am. I'm here for all the people on the seventh floor. You're all equal."

"Except Young Dean, who's more equal."

"Well, no, not except Dean—"

"Shut the fuck up," Wes finally says, too loudly. "You guys are screwing with a good buzz here. But, Jesus Christ, I can always make a new spear, take the damn thing away for all I care," and he emphasizes his point by banging himself in the head with the strings of his tennis racquet. "For fuck's sake, Wagner, why are you wasting your time talking to Chucklehead Charlie? For Christ's sake, man. He's a pinhead."

"I was bored."

"So fill up your day some other way. You will have to learn to fill up days sooner or later."

"What the hell does that mean exactly, Wes?" I'm not in agreement.

"It means it ain't the last time you'll be bored. Life in a wheelchair is fucking boring. What else could it be? I hope there is more than this. It feels like I've been in this hospital for a hundred fucking years already, and I'm sick of it, but there is no *more than this*, so quit fucking looking for it."

"Thanks, I feel better already. Wes, good talk, glad to fucking know you."

"Well, I know something that will make you feel better," says Charlie. I'd almost forgotten he was there until he chirped up.

"Are you still here?" I ask, suddenly sick of discussing my life with him. "Don't you have some counseling to do down the hall or in another part of the hospital where I'm not? Go look for Young Dean's lance. Go save another hapless Quad from himself somewhere else."

"Okay, I can take a hint, but the word is they will put you in an electric chair tomorrow. It'll open up a whole new world for you."

"A whole new world, huh? It's a pretty sad life when an electric wheelchair can open up a whole new world. So don't be disappointed if I don't get all giddy with excitement."

Our little talk finally breaks up because supper is served. Supper (or dinner) takes precedence over anything that might be pending, including a new electric wheelchair. It is the most over-steamed tasteless shit you can imagine, but it signifies one hour before the real good drugs come out. My life was composed of eating and drugs. I would get chicken wings because it was chicken wing day, and it was the one thing they couldn't fuck up. So I forget about the electric wheelchair until I get put into bed an hour later, mind fucked on Demerol, and then despite myself, I get a little excited by the prospect of the little bit of independence an electric wheelchair might afford me.

I am excited and sad. Sad because it is such an unfortunate thing to get excited about.

CHAPTER TWENTY-ONE

MORE ANGER, MORE DENIAL

I'M PLEASANTLY SURPRISED AND ADMITTEDLY more keyed up and thrilled than expected. I've had the electric wheelchair for all of two hours now, and I was supposed to have it back an hour ago.

I'm just not ready to give it up. I've been from one end of the hospital to the other, and although I know that hospitals are probably the most wheelchair-accessible places on Earth, it still feels like I can go anywhere.

Previously, it was a twenty-minute, excruciatingly slow procedure to navigate from the hallway outside my room down to the lounge to get a can of pop or a coffee. I would much rather have gone without at times than go through that particular humiliation. Nurses would pass me like I was standing still. They would pat me on the back, encouraging my efforts, while I grunted and groaned, pushing the chair at about half a mile an hour. My shoulders would burn, and my hands would invariably slip off the rails of the chair, and I would have to push on the rubber wheels themselves to encourage movement out of a wheelchair that should have been mothballed before I was born.

The old crows waiting beside the elevator are all part of the gauntlet to the lounge. They would see me coming, clapping their hands while sporting big toothless gummy grins. I think they were just happy to see someone slower and more feeble than they were. I would save a little extra in the tank for my big finishing kick to the lounge door just to get by the old crows. The big finish had me reaching speeds of about a mile an hour, a pace almost equal to that of a turtle in a flat-out hurry.

But not now. Now I am positively moving along at a gallop. This electric rig can motor along at five miles an hour, but it feels like fifty, and I am flying. I have been running this thing wide open the minute I got the hang of it, which was no easy task.

That morning, when the therapist transferred me to the electric chair, she warned me to keep it on low and, in her words, "Don't get cute." It sounded good until I was out of sight and had a chance to test the limits of my new conveyance. At first I was a little tentative as I refused the seatbelt, but I quickly learned to lean back; that way I could maintain my balance. I held on tight while I cornered, hugging the chair with my elbows, and once my confidence soared, I put it in high, and I've had it in high ever since. I am as happy as a dog with his head out the car's window.

I'm now on the seventh floor, avoiding the therapist who is waiting for me downstairs because I plan to keep this chair. As of this moment, I have no intention of bringing it back. Young Dean has been using it for the last two weeks, and he thinks it is his. It is, in actuality, a demo chair supplied by Quickie, a big name in wheelchairs, and they let the hospital borrow it in the hope that some sorry Quad will become accustomed to their product and buy one. At this moment, the chair is selling itself. They have reached their demographic. I am a captive audience. I cruise in to see Wes, who is listlessly chasing bees around our room with his aluminum racquet, and he suggests I go run over a few of the old crows at the elevator.

"And while you're there, get me a can of pop," he adds as I spin out of the room.

"Aye, aye, and goodbye," I say as I crank it up and spin the wheels as I navigate the corner. I am rewarded with a small squeak, and I imagine I can smell the rubber burning.

It takes me a lot longer than I would like to get a can of pop for Wes because I decide to get myself a cup of evil tasting, freeze-dried coffee, which means filling up a plastic cup, scooping coffee into it, and sticking it in the microwave to heat it to a boil. Then I must put a tray on my lap and put the tasty beverages on the non-slip tray. This procedure would take a walking person with fingers three minutes at most. Instead, it takes me close to ten.

I finally manage to work out the balancing act, and I move a little slower going back, but my confidence returns as I near the room. I can see that Mr. Mawani and his entourage of hopeful inheritors are returning from their brief sojourn at therapy, and the need to impress eclipses the need for caution. I crank up the Quickie 2000 electric wheelchair to maximum power. They have just entered the room, and I intend to squeal around the corner and surprise and astonish everybody in attendance.

All goes well until the coffee and pop start to slip on the non-slip surface, and in my mind's eye, I foresee the likelihood of one or both of them ending up in my lap, and hot coffee in my lap would be a blistered mess.

I release the death grip I've had on the chair with my left elbow, and I make an automatic grab for the hot coffee at the exact moment when I should be executing my pinpoint turn. Unfortunately, I realized my mistake a second too late, and before I could recover, I released the joystick and the wheelchair stopped dead in its tracks. I am now airborne, launched like a human missile going five miles an hour straight at the cinderblock wall.

My knees hit first with a knuckle-crunching, popping sound like someone had stepped on a raw chicken, but I feel nothing. Nothing, at least until my body catches up to my knees. My head rebounds off the unyielding concrete with a dull thud, like smashing a coconut against a rock. There is searing agony in my neck that travels down my shoulders. I wind up in an undignified heap at the bottom of the wall, soaked in hot coffee and pop.

There is a brief moment of white explosive pain until I lose consciousness, and then everything comes slowly back into focus. I see stars—fuck that, I see galaxies. I hear Wes laughing his ass off, I listen to people running, and I blink my right eye repeatedly because it is full of what can only be blood. At first, I try to push and twist myself away from the wall, but the wheelchair effectively traps me because pushing and twisting are two things I no longer do well. So in the end, it's much easier just to give up, wait for help, and watch the blood drip off my nose to form a widening pool on the linoleum floor.

Help arrives quickly. Nurses and a janitor take great pains to stabilize my neck even though I assure everyone involved that my knees have taken the worst of the impact, and aside from the blood, my head feels fine. Miraculously, I still feel nothing in my knees even though I'm confident I've smashed or broken something in there.

I'm gang-lifted back into the electric chair after my rescuers are reasonably sure I haven't broken my neck once again, and from there they unlock the gears and I'm *pushed* back to my bed and gently dropped onto the mattress. They strip my clothes off, and I'm expertly poked and prodded by Monique and Althuna (who look very concerned) for obvious breaks or dislocations until Doctor Dumars appears, and he, in turn, pokes and prods me some more. He has a stern look on his face. It can only mean a grim prognosis.

"My first impression is that you have damaged the patella on your right knee," he intones with some gravity, looking to me for a response, but for the life of me, I can't see where this presents much of a problem. The stars are still there, but they're just background noise, and I can think clearly. I have destroyed or otherwise impaired a body part that has been already rendered useless by a previous condition known as a broken fucking neck. So what possible difference can it make if I have crushed my knees? But I keep that opinion to myself.

"Oh shit, well, I suppose that will set my impending recovery back indefinitely," I say instead.

"Sarcasm aside, it does present a problem. We'll have to X-ray your knee or knees to be certain, but in the interim you'll be put back on a Heparin drip to avoid blood clots, and you'll be confined to your bed until the swelling goes down."

"So, what if the knee is damaged? What are you going to do, fix it?"

He appears to be in deep thought. "Well, we could operate, but that's a decision to be made when we know more." I'm not sure whether *Doctor Doom* understands just what I'm asking. I'm trying to convey to him the idea that my knee is the least of my problems, but I know what he is doing. *Doctor Doom* is treating me. He is handcuffed when it comes to curing the real problem, so he is helping where he can. "Do no harm." I believe that's the doctrine. In the face of overwhelming odds, it's better to concentrate on a small thing that isn't out of his control, if broken knees can be called a small thing.

"And we'll get you all stitched up as good as new, and we'll look after that nasty gash," he continues, and I get a picture of a front-line doctor on a battlefield who has lost all perspective in the face of overwhelming odds. My legs are fucked up heavily, and he's putting a band-aid on my head. I think I have just had a glimpse of a part of Doctor Dumars' personality that was a mystery to me before this mishap. It's not that he never cared; he feels helpless. He is flustered and upset, and he's not sure what to make of me. That will go on my headstone one day. "Randy Edward Wagner lies here, and we're not sure what to make of him."

"Thanks, Doc. A few stitches, and I'll be as good as new, or at least as good as I once was. While I'm waiting, could you get me a little Demerol or Morphine to ease the pain?" Ease the pain, my ass. I still don't feel a thing, save for a minor headache, and I find it strange that I would give just about anything to feel even a little bit of pain for the first time in my life. This "little" bump on the knee further cements the idea entrenched in my brain that the feelings in my legs are not coming back, ever.

Two hours later, one or two X-rays confirm the worst. I have successfully mashed one patella to a pulp and cracked the other one. I receive eleven stitches in my head (call me Franken-Wag), which puts the total of head stitches at a ridiculous number that exceeds my I.Q. However, I'm sure my I.Q. has been steadily dropping since I punched through the sunroof what seems like a lifetime ago. The headaches come and go, but I haven't told Doctor Dumars about them yet. I don't need any more complications. The restaurant will not wait for me, and we still intend to open up on schedule. So suck it up, buttercup.

Worst of all, I'm again confined to my bed, mainlining rat poison to keep my blood thin, so consequently, my spirits are flagging. It feels like I have just taken a giant step backward and caught the big snake in the Snakes and Ladders game. I have landed on Boardwalk without a single five-hundred-dollar bill in my possession with my railroads mortgaged to the hilt. I am still busy thinking of other crisis metaphors when my wife walks into the room, dressed for work at the Keg.

The Keg has figured into my life too much lately. Push comes to shove; they're our competition if we successfully open a Boston Pizza. So it makes me dislike the Keg even more, and although I know this is irrational somewhere deep down, it still makes me irritable and moody.

"Going to work?" I ask in such a way that implies it isn't *working* at all but some restaurant fantasy camp she attends just to get away from the overwhelming oppressiveness of the hospital and me in particular.

"Yes, I'm going to work. Someone has to," my wife replies defensively. Even as she says it, I know she doesn't mean to imply that I'm not pulling my weight and bringing home my share of the family bacon. But sometimes we don't see the forest for the goddamn trees, and harsh words gather momentum like the little rocks that may start small but become substantial ugly boulders.

"I wish I were going to work," I say morosely, kicking a couple more rocks into the landslide.

"So do I," she replies.

"Meaning what? That I'm laying here being lazy by choice?"

"No, not that. Just that, why the fuck did you have to drive to Lethbridge that night? Why couldn't we sleep the night in Calgary and go in the morning? You're always in such a hurry to get somewhere. Now look where you are."

"Where am I?" I challenge.

"You're in a hospital bed, and you're a Quadriplegic."

"You finally figured that out, did you? You finally got it through your fucking head that I'm not going to get any better."

"It sure doesn't look like it, but I'm not in the mood to talk about it right now. I've got to go to work. I'll see you tomorrow." And with that decision, she squeezes my hand and walks out of the room. She almost makes it to the door, neither looking right nor left to acknowledge Wes or Mr. Mawani and his family. They are uncharacteristically subdued and have been whispering back and forth like children in a church before I gather what little wits I have about me and try to salvage some of my dignity.

"Sorry for ruining your fucking life," I yell. It doesn't salvage my dignity, but I get in the last word, and in the end that's all I wanted to do. It does make her stop before she exits out the door completely, and for a second she almost turns before something stops her, and she resolves to keep going. I know without seeing her face that I have callously gut-punched her with my ill-timed comment, and she will be crying by the time she reaches her car. She didn't deserve that, but Wes chirps up before I have a chance to wallow in regret about my parting words.

"Is that a crack in the ice, Mr. Fucking Perfect? Got a little wake-up call, did you? Knock, knock, who's there? Hello, it's the rest of your goddamn fucking life."

"Fuck you, Wes, and know that you are now, without reservation, on the top of my list."

"Yeah, yeah, you and your goddamn list. Maybe in the last life you could've mopped the floor with me, Mr. Muscle Head, but in this life you're shit. You are not even a special Quad, just a run-of-the-mill fucking Quad. You're not walking out of here. You're rolling out the same way you came in. I've heard you say all the right things, and you're probably telling your-self all the right things, but this is the first time I see it finally sinking in that you're not fucking perfect."

"Hey, Wes, did I bug you when your wife or fiancée or whatever the hell she was kicked sand in your face? No. Did I say, 'Hey Wes, Para-loser dickhead, I hope she goes out and fucks the next ignorant, long-haired, wannabe rock star, farm boy look-alike she sees'? No, I didn't say that. Do you know why I didn't say that? I didn't say that because I don't live my life for the sole purpose of making other people's lives hell, you stinking misery vampire. So I keep my mouth shut when I don't have anything positive to add. And just so you know, you're now the first five names on my list. Right up there on top of the list, it reads Wes, Wes, Wes, Wes, and Wes. The first five people I will kick in the nuts when I learn to walk again."

"You still don't get it, do you?" says Wes, visibly shaken. We have both taken our whacks, and we don't feel good about it, but we're not smart enough to quit swinging. Wes still has a point to make, and he won't be sat-isfied until he makes it. He bangs his racquet on the bedrail to emphasize every syllable. "You're a Quad, and you are no fucking better than the rest of us. Get used to it."

"Are you happy now?" I ask him, smiling my best steely, death wish, I-want-to-kill-you smile.

"Yes," he says.

"Good, and you're right."

"Huh?" He doesn't expect this.

"I said you're right, fuckhead. I have been cruising around here imagining that I'm better than the rest of you by virtue of my imaginary big brain and my doting wife. I have set myself apart. I did it unconsciously. That means without thought, reflexively—"

"I know what it fucking means."

"Yeah, right, sorry about that. I guess I'm just trying to put myself at a distance, as if what you guys have contracted is contagious or something. Like I'm going to be a Quad or a Para by association or osmosis if I hang around with you guys long enough. So maybe I think that when I finally do my stretch here on the seventh floor, and I get out in the real world, if I don't act like a Quad or think like a Quad, I won't be a Quad. Do you see what I'm getting at?"

"That's just denial. If it quacks like a duck and fucks like a duck, it's a duck, and it doesn't matter what you want to call it."

"So you think. You just keep spouting your little Farmer Brown homilies and see where it gets you. I'm going with what works for me. I know I'm a Quad, but I don't choose to act like one. Being a Quad is not going to define me."

"You're—"

"And I'm sleeping now, so shut the fuck up."

"You're not sleeping . . . Oh, fuck you, just because you close your eyes, it doesn't mean you're sleeping. You always do that shit. You're in heavy denial."

"Sleeping, fuck you, and fuck denial."

"Fake sleeping."

"Sleeping, and quit banging on my fucking bed with your stupid racquet."

"Not."

"Sleeping heavily now."

"Bullshit, denial, denial, denial. You're going backward."

"Dreaming now. Dreaming you died in your sleep and went to Paraplegic hell." And the last thing I think about before I fall asleep is that the idea of a Paraplegic hell is somewhat redundant.

CHAPTER TWENTY-TWO

BARGAINING, AGAIN

DAY FIFTY-FIVE. THERE IS NO crucial milestone today, save that my rat poison intravenous line is gone, and the danger of blood clots has passed me by again. My knees are no longer the size of cantaloupes, and my head doesn't hurt; small victories, but victories nonetheless.

Yup, I'm feeling good today, even with the blood clot scare. Monique, Pam, and Althuna have transferred me under protest into my wheelchair, the non-electric post-war Edsel, a wheelchair someone should have put to pasture years ago. They make me sit in it for at least two hours daily, and today is no different. Once I am sitting in it semi-comfortably, they then come in and lift me every twenty minutes or so just so my ass gets shifted into another spot and the blood flow isn't compromised. They usually put me in the chair every day around the time they think my wife is visiting because then they don't have to worry about lifting me. I would give up the drugs they are feeding me if I could lift my own ass off the chair. Unfortunately, an inch is a mile on the seventh floor.

My wife and I are talking civilly to each other again. I had my little blow-up, and I'm better. She keeps herself pretty tightly reined in now, but I can sense an irreparable chip in the concrete, for lack of a better term. The bubble has burst might help clarify things. We have both said something we wish we could take back, but both know this is impossible. You can't put the cat back into the bag, and it's not like we have run out of things to discuss, like the hospital. The hospital is a tiny microcosm, and we are getting to know the nurses more like real people, not just people put on the planet to thanklessly indulge whiners. At least we are getting to know Nurse Arlene, with the "great nuts"; Pam, with the pierced ears; and Monique, the French nurse: my wife speaks French, so that was a given. Althuna remains distant, as does the parade of part-time or casual nurses that briefly come up from the third floor, the floor where there were no roommates, where life is easy, and the burnout ratio isn't what it is up here on the seventh. I still get visits from the pretty but plain Nurse Chalmers, and she remains my personal favorite. It is impossible not to get a crush on at least one or more of the nurses, as they are your lifeline, and I have developed a needless crush.

When I was still in my Halo on the seventh floor, Nurse Chalmers came to visit me one morning after her midnight-to-whenever shift, and I bitched about my itchy head. It was just me and my "Halo" that I couldn't scratch, laying here hour after hour. So instead of just patronizing me with platitudes, she grabbed a big garbage pail, put plastic bags around my head and Halo, and she washed my hair. The water sluiced down the plastic bag into the bucket, and she "Head and Shouldered" the shit out of my hair twice. I fell in love twice over; it was the most incredible feeling on the planet. I felt like a grizzly bear might feel that had just rubbed his back on a gnarly tree for ten minutes. It was damned unfortunate that I ever left the third floor, but I understood. They have a couple of ICU types on the third floor, but generally they deal with less severe cases like the broken bones and knee and hip replacement types that get better and leave in a week to go home to their families. The seventh floor is for people sticking around way too long—the severely fucked up are sent to the seventh, and it becomes your new address.

Arlene, Pam, and Monique always *stay* on the seventh floor because they have chosen to do so. Their reasons are their own, and they are varied. Pam, I learned, actually met her husband of three years on the seventh floor. She has stayed here ever since because she prefers to work with spinal cord and brain-injured people, stroke victims, and abandoned old wrinkly people who comprise this floor's main population. This decision seems very weird to me, but she has promised to bring in her husband one day so I can meet him. I don't know what can be accomplished by such a meeting, but I don't voice my reservations, and I try to sound thrilled at the prospect.

Arlene is here because she is second-in-command after the Charge Nurse, and she genuinely likes the seventh floor because she thinks she's making a difference. Word has it that her mother is in a wheelchair, but the reason for this was never made clear. So, the story goes, and goes, and goes. What else are we going to talk about at the end of the day?

Then there's Monique. I don't know how long Monique has been on the seventh, but she's staying now because she is secretly dating Vince the upright Para, who looks like he has the best chance to walk out under his own power. Monique is charming after you get to know her, but she still has trouble pronouncing the letter "H". Wes, in his words, would kill to get a simple blowjob from Monique when he's up and walking again, and he states it daily, but he can't for the life of him understand why she likes a "putz" like Vince the upright Para. It gives Wes what he calls "the faint hope clause" because if a guy like Vince the upright Para can score with a babe like Monique, why shouldn't he be shacking up with Pamela Anderson the day after his release?

Wes and I have never taken each other to task for anything said earlier in the heat of battle. Every day is a battle of some sort, and emotions run very high. Things get said daily that might be taken to heart in the outside world, but nothing sticks in the close confines of institutional living. You develop a Teflon outer coating in the hospital, which hopefully will come in very handy on the outside.

I'm sitting in my chair right now, patiently waiting for my wife to visit. She has planned to attend my therapy session this morning, where we will use a transfer board for the first time. She wants to watch the procedure, so we can both get away from the oppressive atmosphere that pervades the hospital. Adams is coming back to Calgary to take us out for dinner and check on my progress, and she wants to make sure I will be able to get in and out of the car. I reflect for just a second on how simple life used to be, where the idea of getting in and out of a car wasn't a reason for anxiety or concern. Oh, how we take the simple things for granted. I'm betting this won't be the last time I have this thought.

While I'm sitting in my chair trying to lift my arm to shoulder height, finding it very difficult to do so, I chance to look over at the bed recently occupied by the ever-polite Mr. Mawani. It makes me wonder (once again) whether Wes knew the implications of Mr. Mawani's *bed* choice.

Wes convinced him to move to the spot he had vacated after the "incident" with Thomas. I feel that Wes's insistence that Mr. Mawani move was motivated by a lot more than superstition and "it's right close to the bathroom."

I was even getting used to the constant chatter of his doting family, and I was certainly going to miss those East Indian dishes they prepared for him, hoping that he might show them some recognition or favor. Mr. Mawani was probably going to recover from his affliction, which, as it turned out, wasn't Green Beret disease at all but something called Guillain-Barre syndrome that I read up on in the hospital library. It is a disease of unknown etiology blah, blah, blah. It paralyzes a person for a couple of months and can vanish entirely. His family would have been very disappointed to hear about the almost one hundred percent recovery rate. When I approached Mr. Mawani about this, he suggested keeping the secret between us. "A little bit of knowledge can be a belly belly dangerous thing," he said one night when his family left his bedside so the rest of the hospital could sleep. "They all help me belly good and what they know, or do not know, can be a good ting. Perhaps I will be recovering between my God and me, and nobody else thanks belly much." I took the hint and kept my mouth shut. But all said and done; we'll never know whether his recovery was imminent because he didn't stay long enough to let the affliction run its course.

It seems Thomas T. Thomas was not a forgiving soul, and he never could bring himself to forgive Wes for attempting to smother him. I'm almost convinced that he would have eventually forgotten. Still, Wes continued to remind him daily with his constant hazing rituals, but the final straw was the compact discs.

Thomas had a huge collection of compact discs (CDs), from Abba to ZZ Top, with Hank Williams and Garth Brooks in between. When he came out of his coma (and long before Wes tried to smother him), he would plug one CD into his disc player and play that particular disc all day. CDs were a new technological advance, and they became Thomas's touchstone. Each day, he would go to the next one in line. Then, as they were all alphabetized by his mother or himself (the capabilities of brain-injured people were a mystery to me), he would eventually listen to each one in its turn. Then presumably, he was going to start all over again. He was obsessive about his CDs, and even though Thomas had a brain injury, he seemed to know where each was supposed to be. Thomas freaked out if anyone but his mother, or the nurses he deemed worthy, attempted to touch them. Of course, Wes knew this.

On one fateful day, not long after "the incident," Wes opened the bottom portion of Thomas's door—the nurse's station was vacant—and went into Thomas's room. He not only mixed up the alphabetized CDs but also changed the cases on several of them, putting the Tom Petty in the Elton John case or the Shania Twain in the Green Day case. Wes wasn't sure how many he mixed up, but a good portion. He was immensely proud of himself after this little bit of skullduggery.

"I just spent the morning messing with Thomas's mind," he informed me as if this was something new.

"So basically, it's just another day in paradise," I said, half listening, not realizing the repercussions of what this small event would have on hospital life as we knew it. That morning was the catalyst.

The way I see it, when Thomas T. Thomas came back from therapy (there were no music listening devices there), and when he plugged in his CD, he got a different one than he was expecting. Of course, this would have been unacceptable to Thomas since he was obsessive about the order of his CDs. But anyone possessing even rudimentary cognitive skills could figure out the root cause of this and every other problem he had run into since his arrival on the seventh floor.

When I look back on it, someone should have seen it coming. Wes harassed Thomas openly and thoroughly, and everyone had a breaking point, but the only one prepared for the depth of Thomas's hatred was Wes.

Thomas had been improving in leaps and bounds compared to what he was like when I first met him. I understand he still screamed in the night—thankfully in a room where we could no longer hear him—but he could now comprehend simple commands and form sentences, structured or otherwise. He could feed himself, and he could stand up on his shaky, once broken and shattered legs, taking two or three steps at a time with the use of a sturdy wooden cane—a gift from his father—who had been in to see him three times in the two months I had been here.

I don't know if Thomas waited until the nurses' station was vacant or just had a stroke of dumb luck. I would be more inclined to bet on the latter, but at around three o'clock in the morning, he plopped into his wheelchair, rolled up to the door, and simply stood up and reached over the top of the barn door. Of course, the top was always open so the nurses could monitor Thomas's late-night behavior, but they never suspected he could stand up and quickly release the lock on the bottom of the door and push it open.

Once freed from his makeshift prison, it was a small matter to put the cane in his lap and push the wheelchair four doors down to where an unsuspecting Wes slumbered, blissfully unaware of the extent of Thomas's hatred.

Thomas pushed his chair with the help of his right foot. His arms and hands worked, but not in unison. If he insisted on just using his arms, his chair would get off course and eventually go in circles. His right foot remedied this problem. He used it almost as a tiller as he propelled his wheelchair backward, always backward, using his right foot to push, dragging his left foot to further assist him in steering a straight and true course. It was his dragging foot I heard that night as he piloted his wheelchair four doors down and into the room inhabited by Wes, Mr. Mawani, and myself.

He was wearing his cross-trainers, versatile runners, useful in therapy and perfect for a late-night foray into enemy territory. But ultimately, the squeak of his dragging left sneaker on the linoleum woke me up before he ever came through the door. If the privacy curtain had been open, I would have known who it was, and his intentions might have become clear before it was too late.

I was half asleep, and my subconscious tracked the squeaking sound as it came down the hall and entered the room. I was half in and half out of my latest suffocation dream, where I consistently woke up feeling either like I was drowning or someone was holding a plastic bag over my head.

My drug of choice was still Demerol when I could get it. They were trying to wean me off my dependency, giving it to me every five hours instead of four.

The first true inkling I had that Thomas T. Thomas was in our room, besides the squeaking running shoe, was the sound of him humming and grunting as he purposefully struggled to his feet and took the last couple of painfully slow steps toward Wes's bed. That is to say, the bed where Wes used to sleep.

The bed was now claimed by Mr. Mawani on Wes's insistence that the bed on the *other* side of the room (Bob's old bed) was cursed, and that this new one was "right close to the bathroom" and was prime real estate.

The first meaty THUNK of the sturdy wooden cane hitting flesh brought me fully awake. The second meaty THUNK caused me to shout Thomas's name aloud, and the third meaty THUNK told me in no uncertain terms that I was too late to do anything but let the drama play itself out. Unfortunately, I couldn't reach the damned ripcord. It had fallen off the bed and was stuck behind my head.

Thomas was killing Wes. At least in Thomas's mind, he was killing Wes. Thomas had no idea that an old Hindu man named Mr. Mawani had taken up Wes's old bed and Wes had moved to the space vacated by Thomas.

I don't know how many times the cane came down, more times than I care to remember. It was a case of overkill. I prefer to think Mr. Mawani didn't suffer at all, and the first blow knocked him senseless.

As it turned out, Wes was the one that eventually pulled the ripcord to summon the nurses. By then, it was a moot point as the nurses didn't arrive until Thomas had wholly exhausted himself and sat back down in the wheelchair. He was starting to back out of the room, his mission a roaring success, his cross-trainer squeaking on the linoleum, when the first nurse arrived on the scene, followed by two more. I could hear their voices. Mr. Mawani was quickly wheeled away. Every nurse on the seventh floor was spurred into action by then. I just lay there, stoned. The morning came, and when they pulled my cloth curtain open, Mr. Mawani's bed was absent, as was Mr. Mawani. I never saw him again.

CHAPTER TWENTY-THREE

ANGER AGAIN, SOME BARGAINING

MY WIFE AND I ARRIVED at therapy, and she had this big smile plastered to her face—which had been there since day forty-six when I had given myself over to the inevitable that Quadriplegia loomed over my future. Now I find the easiest way to carry on each day is to think about my next milestone, any minor or seemingly insignificant change. Anything is progress.

According to the therapist, today we gravitate to the transfer board, a significant milestone that will make my life easier by degrees I cannot comprehend. But it is vital for me because it will get me out of the hospital for the first time, which is incentive enough.

I would gladly crawl over broken glass and razor wire to get a reprieve from the sheer drudgery of the hospital. I was at odds with Wes and wished I could wipe the smug smile off his face. However, I heard through the grapevine that Mr. Mawani did survive. Thomas missed his head but connected with subsequent blows to his body, so Guillain-Barre syndrome was the least of his problems. I tried not to think about it. I was getting real good at putting myself first, one step at a time.

The first hurdle is getting the transfer board under my butt, a butt that, at times, seems filled with lead weights and then stapled to the chair. I am still a long way off from lifting myself off the seat of the wheelchair. I'm assured this will get easier in time. Jenny is my physiotherapist, and she is built like a Russian powerlifter. She can pick me up and transfer me herself by putting my knees in her lap, picking me up by the shoulders, and pivoting me onto the mat. She would crush anyone I know in "midget bowling" if that were an official sport.

I have pulled the chair up next to the king-size workout mat to lift my ass off the chair's seat. The seat of the wheelchair was the same height, and I only had to raise myself one inch to get the board underneath me. I am being encouraged to lift as I've never lifted before.

"Imagine your ass is filled with helium," says Jenny, which causes me to laugh instead of think about the lift. I have both hands on the chair's wheels, and I am pushing down with all my might, but the triceps muscles I once took for granted will not be awakened, and I have not budged my butt an inch. I try to keep the frustration off my face, but it is painfully evident.

"Let me lift him," suggests my wife, who it seems has no capacity for watching me struggle. Although her smile shows some wear, she cannot stop thinking back to a time when everything came easy, where the simple act of lifting my ass off a chair was no more complicated than tying my shoes or brushing my teeth, neither of which I can do anymore.

"We're going out for dinner tonight, so we don't have the luxury of time," she adds, again insinuating that I'm not trying hard enough. There is nothing I would like better than to lift my ass a couple of inches off this stinking wheelchair, but try as I might, I just can't get any air.

"Okay, lift him," says Jenny, sighing audibly. She seems more impatient with my wife than she is with me, judging by the tone of her voice.

"I'll do it by myself eventually," I say, more to myself than to anyone else, as my wife grabs underneath my arms and proceeds to lift me clear of the chair, all one hundred fifty pounds of the *new* me.

I realize that there is nothing more cumbersome, more inexorably heavy, and more relentlessly awkward than a dead body. Hence the term "dead weight" and all that it implies. Unfortunately, my body is now all of the above, dead, inexorably heavy, and completely uncooperative.

My wife lifts, and all she manages to do is pull my t-shirt out of my sweatpants and skid my butt two inches to the right. Great for relieving pressure but useless when inserting a transfer board.

Finally, Jenny lifts me by bending me forward over her shoulder and heaving me upward with her legs. In this way, we get the board half underneath me, and I am left alone to move my ass along the board and onto the mat. Again, it's a simple procedure in theory, but it sounds a lot easier than it proves to be.

I end up falling over sideways, and the therapist and my wife barely save me from going face-first into the side of the therapy bed. My wife grabs a handful of my shirt, and Jenny sticks her shoulder under my chin and pushes up, almost choking me in the process. Even worse, all this thrashing around caused the condom catheter to slip off the shaft of my useless dick. So now, I'm leaking urine all over my sweatpants and the seat of the wheelchair.

"Fucking lousy rotten condom catheters," I say, for about the hundredth time, as Jenny pushes me back into the chair and secures me there as my wife yanks out the transfer board. Condom catheters are designed very poorly, and although preferable to getting catheterized every two hours, they never stay adequately attached. If I had a ten-inch dick they might work, but I don't.

Therapy is over for the day, and my wife pushes me back upstairs to the seventh floor, where I can get washed and reattached to the drainage tube. I'm ever so glad I can't see her face because the smile that she has tried so arduously to maintain would be replaced by a severe look of defeat that wouldn't do either one of us any good to acknowledge.

CHAPTER TWENTY-FOUR

DENIAL, ONE LAST TIME, HOPEFULLY

I'M SITTING IN MY WHEELCHAIR when Adams arrives later in the afternoon, and we spend two hours catching up on daily events and mutual friends. We tiptoe around anything to do with hospital life, but it becomes a big elephant in the room that we cannot ignore forever. The elephant represents all of the days of pure hell spent in this goddamn hospital, but I still try to put a good slant on it because who likes a whiny, complaining Quad?

I tell him about Bob dying quietly for no apparent reason. He didn't know Bob. Hell, I didn't know Bob. It just seems like a small victory that I have outlived him. Adams sagely nods like it was inevitable. Adams is good at sagely nodding his head. I tell him about the thrashing of Mr. Mawani, leaving nothing out and embellishing freely. He tries not to laugh, but it is hard to stay serious with Wes chuckling away like some demented James Bond villain right across the room.

Wes has never claimed any responsibility for the caning of Mr. Mawani. He insists it is a fluke that Thomas T. Thomas escaped custody that night and walloped Mr. Mawani into an unrecognizable lump. Wes insists he never saw it coming, only I know that behind the redneck, prejudiced, fucked up façade, Wes is genuinely a cowardly, devious little shit that hates the rest of the entire world and is not capable of accepting responsibility.

I fill Adams in on all the nurses I have met and all the other Quads and Paras that make up the known seventh-floor universe, and I even surprise myself at how pleasant I'm making it all sound. It never even occurs that I haven't said a single thing about myself in the entire two hours until Adams points it out.

"So, how are you progressing?" he finally asks when I have run out of funny stories (and the unfunny ones) about other people.

"Progressing well, thank you. I suppose I'm right on schedule," I declare.

"On schedule for what? What does 'on schedule' mean?"

"For my eventual release in January of the next year."

"That's about five months from now," he says, as if I haven't done the math backward and forwards more times than I can count.

"It takes seven to nine months to process a Quad."

"It sounds like an assembly line."

"You got that right. In a sense, we are being processed in increments. First you learn to walk, and then you learn to run. It would be a fuck of a lot easier if I could learn to quit running into walls, literally and figuratively."

"Bad analogy," he says, failing to see the humor in my last comment. "So, you're telling me that you have at least six or seven months to go before you get out?"

"Think of it as Quad School. I have to take the basic classes that prepare me for life outside the institution. It's not something you can rush. I couldn't even lift my arm off the bed three weeks in. Now I can at least do that, and I can sit in a wheelchair for five hours at a time. It sure doesn't sound like much, but it beats the alternative, which is no improvement at all."

"You're saying all the right things," he says, shaking his head, "but it sounds more like you're reading it off a cue card. This shit has to suck a lot more than you're letting on."

"Okay, it sucks ass. Is that what you want to hear?"

"Don't tell me what I want to hear. Tell me how you're doing without all the bullshit and the obvious denial."

"Who taught you that word? My wife?"

"She might have mentioned it."

"Well, fuck her and fuck you. I am not in denial. Everyone else is."

"You tell him, Wagner," says Wes, who can't help but hear. He could at least pretend he isn't listening, which is the polite thing to do, but it's Wes; privacy is not his strength.

"And especially fuck you too, Wes. Come on, Adams, push me down to the cafeteria or outside if it's not too hot. I'm feeling a little claustrophobic."

"Hey, no argument here. This place sucks. It makes me queasy just being here," and with that, Adams gets behind me and steers me out of the room and towards the elevators. We don't talk as we go by the aged murder of crows gathered at the elevator waiting for the day their turn comes to be pushed somewhere, anywhere significant. Instead, they grin toothlessly and watch as we pass, openly envious of our youth and purpose. It makes me think about how we haven't progressed as far medically as we might think we have. Sure, we can now keep people alive indefinitely, but to what purpose? Most people aren't living healthier, just longer, and in some cases, longer than necessary.

Soon, we'll be giving ninety-year-olds heart transplants just to give them another five years on the planet. Where does it end?

"Doesn't that smell get to you at all?" asks Adams, intruding on my deep thoughts.

"What smell?" I say. I'm trying to remember when I smelled anything that didn't smell like a hospital.

"It's like the smell of death and piss, covered up with disinfectant and deodorizers."

"It's funny you should say that. I remember thinking that when I first got to the seventh floor. I guess I've gotten used to it. Sad but true. It always smells like this. It even gets in your clothes."

"Yeah, now that you mention it, it did smell bad from day one, but we were all a little freaked out, to say the least, when we first came to see you. Bignell and Shea still have trouble talking about it. It was just so surreal. You have a picture in your mind of what it's going to be like, how you're going to look, and then you make it even worse just in case, and you find out it's worse than you could ever imagine."

"So was it worse than you could ever imagine? Now that you've had time to digest it."

"I guess so, but after you think of the alternative, which is you being dead, it doesn't seem so bad."

"I hear ya. You're playing the 'What's Better Sweepstakes' without knowing the game. Is being wheelchair-bound for life better than being dead? I think my friends, family, and possibly my wife are in denial. Not me."

"Enough with denial already," Adams says, sounding a little exhausted. "Let's talk about something else."

"Like what? We're in a hospital. A hospital is the personification of denial, anger, bargaining, and depression, presumptuously leading to acceptance. It's drilled into my fucking head daily, pardon the language, but you can't make a silk purse from a sow's ear."

Our conversation stops as we eventually get in line at the cafeteria. I go for the apple juice. Adams gets a cup of coffee and a doughnut filled with blue sticky paste artificially altered to resemble the flavor of blueberries. The hot food smells good, and it even looks good through the plastic windows: steaming trays of chicken and roast beef with gravy and potatoes that still look like potatoes, not freeze-dried mush. Green vegetables that aren't wilted into submission. Real food, food that would usually be at my mercy, but my appetite just isn't there.

"Are you sure you don't want some chicken or something?" asks Adams.

"Nope. I'll save myself. I hear you're taking me out for dinner tonight, and I'm keeping my options open."

"That's not for another three or four hours, and you could stand to gain a few pounds. It looks like you've lost a lot of weight."

"Apple juice now, beer, wine, and seafood later, in that order."

"Suit yourself," he says, mimicking what has become one of my many new mottos. Yessiree, adages to live by, "Suit yourself," and of course, "Don't sweat the small stuff," and my personal favorite, "One step at a time." I fucking hate the platitudes, but they're unavoidable.

We find a table in the back because I don't like people much. Not lately anyway. They are all so unaware of how much their everyday lives annoy me. They so nonchalantly grip their coffee cups, use their knives and forks, cross their feet, stretch their arms above their heads, and then get up and walk away like they haven't done anything special. I know it's not normal to think like this, but these thoughts come unbidden, and I could not stop them from coming any more than I could stem the tide.

I'm more interested in the afflicted people that pop up, like little black raisins in white rice, dispersed around the hospital cafeteria. As we talk, I look around at the people less fortunate than me, and from them I gather strength. Like Wes, I have inadvertently become a "misery" vampire. It is a sad day.

"Where do you want to go for dinner?" Adams asks, unaware that I am soaking up misery with every breath I take, gathering power and perspective. I bend down and sip from the straw stuck in my apple juice, nodding at a younger fellow two seats away who has to get his juice lifted to his lips. I spot a girl no older than me with a Halo on like the one I used to wear being spoon-fed some soup, and I wonder why I haven't seen her before. Maybe she hasn't graduated up to the seventh floor yet. "You don't know what you're missing, lady," I say to myself.

"Pardon," says Adams.

"What?" I say.

"What am I missing?" he asks, confused.

"Did I say that out loud?" I smile. "I guess I did. Perhaps I should go back upstairs for a nap before you take my wife and me out for dinner. And by the way, I want to go to The Cannery. It will be the first meal I've had outside the hospital, and I want it to be good. Damn the expense."

"Don't worry," he says. "It's my treat. Well, it's Jim and George's treat." It makes me feel good that the head office at Boston Pizza hasn't forgotten about me. They rented a T.V. that I can watch quietly at night, and no one else has one of those. Jim Treliving and George Melville are the most accessible company heads I've ever dealt with. But my mind shifts back to our outing. I'm already thinking lobster and crab.

"Even better," I say, "because I honestly don't know if I could afford it. Money doesn't mean anything in the hospital, and I have no idea how much I have." I think about that on the push back to the room through the sterile off-white hallways. I honestly haven't thought about personal finances once since I've been in the hospital. My wife has to work at the Keg to make ends meet, but is that enough? I don't know. When I crashed the truck, we were barely getting by. We are insured, but to what degree?

The price of the truck, I suppose? There are working days lost never to be recovered. It puts too many scary thoughts into my head, too many scenarios to comprehend. So instead, I will concentrate on the next small milestone and pretend that the rest will take care of itself in time.

CHAPTER TWENTY-FIVE

DENIAL, ONE MORE TIME, AND ANGER

THE NAP REJUVENATES ME. I feel good when Adams comes and picks me up. Surprisingly enough, I am damn hungry. Weird since it has been a long time since I felt hungry. In one of those large informative medical books, I had read somewhere that Quads cannot feel hunger because of the C5 and C6 vertebrae gap.

I saw it on my X-ray. Plain as day, there is a gap that will not heal and cannot be bridged. Because of this gap, all of the triggers that make me feel hungry are destroyed. They are on the old synapse back burner. All the usual commands and response prompts that my brain sends out to my body fall off the edge of the "gap" and get lost somewhere in that chasm between the damaged or pinched area of my spinal cord.

I'm not sure I buy into the hunger thing all the way. Indeed, I haven't felt hungry in the hospital, and who would with the boiled, steamed, and pureed crap they try to pass off as food around here, but I still think I would feel hungry if there was something worth eating. But I have noticed some other glaring changes aside from not feeling hungry, and it definitely has something to do with the all-important fucking "gap." For example, I can no longer sweat like regular people. One night, I discovered that. They had to pack me in ice when I had a fever and bring in several fans to cool me down. Finally, I peaked at 104 degrees, but there wasn't a bead of sweat on my brow. It's like I was burning up inside, but I was cool and dry as a cucumber outside.

That was a weird discovery I filed away for later, because if I ever get around to sitting out in the sun on a hot, humid day, I would be prone to heatstroke without the ability to sweat. So there's just one more goddamn thing to file away for later, among the already numerous things I've had to file away for future reference. In addition, of course, I have discovered that I can no longer sneeze, cough, shit, breathe, and shout like ordinary people, but I learned these lessons quickly, and I have filed them away in my memory under, "You're a fucking Quad, man. Deal with it."

Maybe I'm just hungry by rote, a memory response, a Pavlovian dog thing. I am salivating because I know that the steak, seafood, and wine will taste good. I picked an expensive restaurant with a reputation for fine cuisine. My sense of taste is just fine. It might even be sharper; since I have lost so many of my other senses, it would only stand to reason that the remainder would naturally become more acute. I can't wait to put this theory to the test.

But first, there is the dreaded transfer. The big boat of an automobile that has replaced the truck I destroyed pulls up to the curb where Adams has pushed me, and the door swings open. It is here that we hit our first snag. Adams and my wife are both standing by the open door, waiting for something magical to happen, as if they can get me into the car by just thinking about it. I help them out by trying to levitate, but I fail miserably. I suck at levitating.

"Well, don't just stand there," I say, "take control and push the chair up close to the seat. We'll have to give this transfer board a try eventually."

"I could just lift you," Adams suggests.

"No way, let's do it by the book. Sooner or later, I will have to use this thing. So, let's make it sooner."

"But you can't lift your ass off the chair," says my wife. "How can we get the transfer board underneath you if you can't get airborne?"

"Defeatist talk," I say, and I will have none of that. It is false bravado, again. I don't know how this will go, but I'm hoping for the best. "Push me close to the car seat on an angle, and I'll give it my best shot. Then, it's time to get this show on the road." Although he does what he is told, Adams doesn't honestly know what to expect and looks understandably hesitant.

Once I was beside the car and the board was positioned for insertion under my ass, I lifted an inch and felt good about it as my wife jammed that board underneath me. I give a mighty grunt, which, in reality, is not that mighty at all, but it does serve to inject a shot of adrenaline into my body, and I lift for all I'm worth while at the same time I bend forward at the waist. Unfortunately, the bending thing turns out to be a monumental miscalculation.

I succeed in launching myself face-first right into the space underneath the glove box, where luckily the car seat breaks my fall just enough so that my face doesn't meet the floor mat. It is an uncomfortable position to be in, and it is a full ten to fifteen seconds before either Adams or my wife jumps forward to help pull me back up. I make a note to myself to apprise the onlookers and helpers of my intentions before acting on them. My pride is the only thing damaged. I'm hoisted backward into roughly the same position I started from, sitting precariously on a transfer board.

In the end, Adams goes behind the chair. He lifts me under the arms, and my wife lifts me under my knees. In this fashion, my legs are successfully stuffed into the car. Then a brief but frantic wrestling match ensues as Adams tries to stuff the rest of my body in behind my legs. Finally, the chair is whisked away, and with my wife pushing from the side and Adams utilizing his right knee, the wrestling match is won after a fashion, and I finally arrive inside the automobile. I am half undressed and damn near exhausted, but I am undaunted as I try to look on the bright side. We have completed our first transfer without disturbing the condom catheter, and we are ready to carry on gamely.

"That could have been easier," says Adams, sweating and looking frazzled.

"Could have been harder too," I point out. My wife says nothing. I decide not to push it. It is so good to be outside the hospital that the botched transfer is quickly forgotten, and I look around like I have never seen Calgary before. It looks wonderful. The trees and shrubs and plants are in full flower. The reds look redder, and the blues and yellows look vibrant and alive. The sweet smell of honeysuckle is everywhere. Summer is in full swing, and I almost missed it while gathering dust in the bleak hospital room.

Either Calgary has changed or my perspective has, and if I were a betting man, I would bet on my perspective being the culprit. The smells, the emotions they invoke, the sweet smell of a season that I almost missed. Summer is winding up, and I feel fortunate beyond words to finally get away from hospital life's oppressiveness.

We pass a slo-pitch softball game in one of the parks near the hospital, and I remember my own experiences with an acute sense of longing. The long, slow, lazy afternoons that made up the slo-pitch tournaments I used to participate in pretty much weekly. It was a ritual that would start on a Friday night under the lights and end late on a Sunday afternoon as the sun sank behind the mountains. The oiled leather smell of the baseball gloves mixed with the coconut aroma of sunscreen. After the game, you had to drink the ice-cold beer in the beer garden fast before the sun touched it and took the condensation off the plastic cup. The easy camaraderie, the exaggerated importance of the last play you were involved in, the bragging rights, and the errors are quickly forgotten after that fourth or fifth cold beer. It was all a part of the weekend. I missed that with an almost palpable ache that hollowed me out and squeezed my throat, making it hard to swallow. It made me grit my teeth, and it was all I could do to hold back the tears. I was once more acutely aware of my loss. It sucked all the air out of me, and I hit the side of the door in frustration. I am so definitely going to get drunk tonight.

"You okay there, Wag?" Adams asks, breaking the spell and bringing me back to the present. It makes me wonder if I'll be like this from now on. Whether my future will be filled with grim, pathetic, wool-gathering moments. Brief flashes of past glories and lost opportunities mixed with maudlin memory-lane crap that served me no good and danced me back and forth through a life I had to leave behind far too young. It is too much to think about, and it is easier to concentrate on the present. So, I'll be glad when we arrive at The Cannery.

We get there, and I swallow all the advice I might want to impart, which is hard for me, and I let Adams and my wife formulate a plan. They assemble the wheelchair, dragged out of the trunk in pieces, and Adams places it two paces away from the car.

"What we're going to do here, Wag," he explains, "is lift your body out of the car and swing you into your wheelchair. I'll take your upper body, lifting under your arms, and she'll take your legs. It will be a quick lift, and before you can say 'Bob's your uncle,' we'll plunk you in the chair." I laugh to myself. In Wagner's new world, "Bob" is everyone's uncle. Such a silly but apt parable in so many ways. It is a good, solid plan. However, it might have worked if someone hadn't forgotten to put the brakes on the wheelchair.

They lift me out and take two ungainly steps toward the chair, and it looks pretty good until my hip hits the nearest armrest, which they should have removed, and the chair skips away a couple of feet out of reach. That's when things start to fall apart. Instead of putting me back into the car and starting over, they opt to chase the wheelchair. It is a wrong decision, and once you decide to pursue it, there is no turning back. So, in true Keystone Cop fashion, they bump and track the wheelchair ten feet across the parking lot while I say "Bob's your uncle" every time I can get a breath, which I'm informed, more than once, isn't fucking helping.

In the end, I am left sitting in the gravel parking lot, still only about two or three feet away from the chair. My shirt hiked up to my chin, and my pants were almost down to my knees. It seems every transfer involves undressing and redressing after each attempt. Surprisingly enough, the condom catheter stays taped around my dick, and they roll me over a few times in the gravel until I am once again dressed and ready for action.

First, Adams sits beside me in the gravel parking lot to catch his breath, and he holds me up against him while my wife looks at the errant wheelchair with murder in her eyes. The wheelchair sits stoically beside us, unaware of the trouble it has caused. It is much like a skittish horse that prances away just as you're preparing to swing your leg over its back, and then after you've cursed it blue, it goes back to quietly munching grass as if you never existed.

On try number two, after I am first warned never to say "Bob's your uncle" again under threat of imminent death, the wheelchair is brought right beside me, the brakes set and the armrest removed. These factors alone help immensely, and I'm plunked into the wheelchair as initially promised, but not before my shirt is once again hiked up to my neck. I make another note to myself to perhaps get some tie-downs like hockey players have that prevent your uniform from coming over your head. However, at this point so many strangers have seen me partially clothed that my modesty is no longer a burning concern.

After resting, Adams pushes the wheelchair through the gravel, a feat only accomplished by putting the chair in a wheelie position and balancing the chair on the back wheels as we make forward progress. Adams looks like he has run a marathon, and he could use a shower by the time we arrive at the entrance to the restaurant. And what an entrance it is.

"Did anyone think to call ahead?" I ask.

"Not me," says Adams.

"Me neither," admits my wife, who sighs audibly and looks close to tears. This latest wrinkle might unhinge her and send her screaming into the night, but she turns on me instead because, in her reality, I should have been the one to think of phoning ahead to check the accessibility of the damn restaurant.

"Okay, okay, I should have thought of it. Quit looking at me like that. I'm new at this. It's the first time in my fucking entire life I ever had to think about what 'wheelchair accessible' might mean."

"This is not wheelchair accessible," Adams points out needlessly.

"Thanks, Adams. I'll file that for future reference, just in case it might slip my mind that I'm not about to climb up a flight of twelve steps."

"Thirteen," he says.

"Thirteen, fourteen, six, one, whatever. Unless you guys lift me up this flight of stairs, I'm eating seafood in the parking lot. At this point, I'm getting into the restaurant, or the goddamn restaurant will have to come out to me."

"I'll go get help," says my wife. "There's got to be a few waiters or diners or somebody who can help. You know, you're not easy to lift," she adds, again unnecessarily.

"I kind of gathered that in the parking lot," I say, a little too sarcastically, which gets me a scathing look before she climbs the stairs with the greatest of ease and enters the restaurant. "Bitch," I mutter under my breath.

"Come on," says Adams, "this can't be easy for her."

"What, and it's easy for me? Think about it. It's my first fucking time out of the hospital, and everything is a little exaggerated, made a little worse just because it's uncharted territory. We all have to relax, go with it a little, and treat it as an adventure. We're going down the rapids, and we keep hitting waterfalls, so you have to get out and do a little portaging. It's not the worst thing that can happen. After you get around the fucking waterfalls, you put the canoe back in the water, and you go merrily, merrily, merrily, merrily down the fucking stream." I'm getting pissed off and trying not to become discouraged.

"When did you start swearing so much?" asks Adams.

"Since I broke my neck, how the hell do I know?" Again, I snap. Since the death of my legs, it seems. Blaspheming and swearing now come naturally. I've got a lot of pent-up emotional angst to deal with lately.

"If it fucking feels good, stay with it," he says, shrugging.

"Yeah, that's what I thought too." I notice that we are both staring fixedly at the stairs as if we might somehow straighten them out by the sheer force of will. I forego another opportunity to test my levitation skills, although that would be so cool. Voop, up we go, mission accomplished. "You think this shit gets any easier?" I finally ask.

"I sure fucking hope so," he says just as my wife comes out of the double door with what looks like the entire staff of the Cannery restaurant. They are burly youthful-looking fellows, and before you can say, "Bo Diddley," they have picked me up and danced me up the stairs. I make another note to remember that asking for help is a good thing, an excellent thing.

The entire restaurant experience turned out to be better than I could have hoped for in my imagination. I try a little bit of everything. I savor the lobster and the shrimp and almost drink the garlic butter out of the little heated dish. The steak is a little grainy and challenging, but I think this is partly because I can't chew very well. Chewing hurts my jaw and, by association, the back of my head and, ultimately, my damaged neck, but everything tastes so fresh and succulent. I gladly take a little pain and eat enough to feed a family of four for a week.

The only big disappointment is the beer and wine. The beer is strong and bitter, tasting a lot like it did when I was a kid when I used to sneak a beer from my dad's basement and drink it in the bush. Adams and I would both screw up our faces and wonder how adults could stomach the vile stuff, but beer went on to become one of life's greatest pleasures through perseverance. How could the fates be so cruel as to take that pleasure away? Beer has never let me down before. The wine also tastes way more potent and acidic than I remembered. I eventually have to order a bottle of Black Tower, a sweet little German number that no wine snob would lower himself to sampling. I used to drink that stuff back in grade school. It makes me wonder how much alcohol in all its forms is an acquired taste, and one that is easily un-acquired in no time flat—well, about fifty-some days by my reckoning.

I shall have to persevere, it seems, and persevere I do. I am heroic in my quest to persevere. I manage to get through the entire bottle of Black Tower, and after the third beer, it almost starts to taste good again, but I'm running short of perseverance, and I decide to have a coffee to make sure *they* still taste good, and a second one to make sure the first one wasn't a fluke.

The tab is enormous. I am only too happy to let Adams pay this tab, and I don't even glance at the bill and fumble around with my non-existent wallet offering to get the tip or some such thing. He doesn't seem to mind, and I understand when he breaks out the corporate credit card and puts it on the bill.

"Head office of the Boston Pizza Corporation wants to take care of this one," he tells me happily because the tab is legendary. Moreover, Adams and I are historically good at running up the company credit card. Ah, the good old days.

"Good," I say happily, satisfied, "and remember to thank Jim and George personally for me. It's great to see they haven't forgotten me." I suddenly feel essential, and my eyes water again. It's the fucking drugs. They take away my inhibitions.

"They know you're here," Adams assures me. "They're pulling for you to open the Boston Pizza in Airdrie right on schedule."

My wife smiles at this. She has been strangely quiet during the meal, and only the mention of Jim and George of Boston Pizza fame brings her back into the conversation. She has a soft spot for both of them. They initially hired her during Expo '86 in Vancouver. They picked her to open the Boston Pizza on the Expo site, and she was the one who initially hired Adams to be a line cook or some such thing. The ripples from that particular rock in the pond are still spreading out and touching our lives today. Adams met his wife at the very same Boston Pizza. He is now the head-office kitchen manager in charge of getting new franchises like ours up and running, and he travels to Boston Pizzas all over the country representing head office. Boston Pizzas sprang up like weeds after Expo. We would have never conceived of owning a franchise ourselves if it wasn't for the blessings of the two benevolent owners named Jim and George, who, with the help of a guy called Bernie, got us fixed up with our new partners and gave us a chance to be owner-managers.

I'm gathering wool, but this huge responsibility is never far from my mind as I go off to therapy each day and try to "be all I can be" (that expression still makes me gag) so that I might still contribute to the opening process. The little extra stuff makes up the fabric of your life that keeps you going to therapy every day.

After Adams pays the tab, a strange lethargy almost overwhelms me. I am suddenly exhausted beyond reason. The booze has kicked in, and it's hard to keep my eyes open. My energy reserves are tapped, and my back, despite the alcohol, is getting stiff and sore. It seems I'm going to have to work on my endurance. Nevertheless, after all the initial screw-ups, it has been a great outing, and we are much more relaxed about the prospect of the trip back to the hospital. Not wholly comfortable, just more relaxed.

But we are again faced with the monumental problem of navigating the thirteen stairs. Not so massive an undertaking as it was a couple of hours ago because what goes up must come down, and it has to be a little easier each time you do it. My wife rounds up another three waiters and a busboy, and with Adams helping and my wife giving instructions, we are down the stairs and into the car with little difficulty. With this outing being my first as a Quad, it's hard to compare it to anything, but I have learned that people, in general, are only too happy to help if they get a little instruction. It's a valuable lesson to learn.

CHAPTER TWENTY-SIX

ANGER, ALWAYS ANGER, IT NEVER LEAVES

IT IS DAY SEVENTY-SIX OR seventy-seven; I'm not sure which. Time has no place in a hospital, but I insistently keep mentally ticking the days away. Sometimes, days blend into each other, as I'm sure they must if you were in prison or stranded on an island in the middle of the Pacific. Believe it or not, either one of those scenarios seems preferable to my current situation. I can't even put a scratch on a wall or an X on a calendar.

A typical day has me awake at seven-thirty after eight hours of fitful sleep, interrupted by three turns and one drug fix. Every day at around seven a.m., a nurse opens the privacy curtain, checks my intravenous line, and adds a bag of mystery ingredients, depending if you have a blood clot or a bladder infection. I am finding out first-hand that these two things are a common occurrence. Sometimes she takes some blood, and sometimes not. I can sleep through the entire process.

If it's a commode day or a bowel day, I get a suppository at seven-thirty and sit over a toilet by eight. Seated over a toilet happens three times a week, and I no longer fight it, as it is just part of the routine. I don't try to translate this into life on the outside. "One step at a time," I remind myself. Next, depending on which day it is, I get dressed and head down to the therapy room, or I get a shower. On a shower day, you get trundled down the hall on a rickety commode chair, buck naked or with a towel in your lap, and you end up in a tiled room, where you're sprayed down and soaped up much like a dusty old car going through the car wash, rinsed, toweled off and *then* you are sent to therapy. Everything you do, every breath you fucking take, centers on therapy.

Therapy is what makes my little hospital world go around. How much weight can you pull, push, or drag on a given day? How often can you propel your creaky post-war wheelchair around the little indoor track, or how long can you tread water until you sink like a big rock? That part is a big learning curve. Just forget that you could swim like a fish before breaking your neck. That was a memory, and this is my new life. Now you need little preschool orange water wings attached to your upper arms to keep your head above the water in a pool barely more significant than some of the hot tubs they have around today. The swimming portion of therapy is the only physical therapy aspect I enjoy, but let us not forget about occupational therapy.

You could call it what it is, Survival 101, or how to try and exist in a new world you were never meant to live in, a strange new world. In occupational therapy, you get to do mundane tasks that were not difficult before. You do this while trying to maintain some semblance of dignity. In occupational therapy, I am trying to learn to write again. I am putting a pen or a pencil in my dead useless fingers and attempting to form letters on paper. It is worse than being back in grade school, where you repeatedly print the letter "A" five thousand times until you get it right. I have put the pen in between my fingers in an interlocking grip, I have turned my hand around backward and used the other hand to steady the pen, and I've used my mouth once in frustration, gripping the pen in my teeth. I have done everything, save sticking the pen up my ass and moving my body back and forth, but my As still looks like little stickmen caught in hurricane-force winds. The things I took for granted before this now become the focus of my new life.

Today in "Occ Therapy," they gave me a can opener and a fake can. It's empty. It's as if an actual, real can of soup or beans could be lethal in the wrong hands, and they stood back while I tried to "problem-solve." Anything you accomplish in "Occ Therapy" they call problem-solving. In the end, I started slamming the can and the opener against the table in a two-handed overhead ax chop. In retrospect, maybe it's a good thing they gave me a fake soup can with nothing in it. It takes me only ten minutes to decide that anything in a can is off my list. I slam the can into dented metal bits and cut my hand, but I don't give a shit. The can of nothing becomes all fucked up and twisted, just like me, and the therapist waits around patiently while I take out my frustrations.

When therapy is over, you push your sorry tired ass upstairs and get another drug fix and attempt to take an afternoon nap or go up to the smoking balcony on the eighth floor. There you can watch Wes, Carl, and Scott get so stoned they forget, for just a minute, that they're stuck in a hospital, being institutionalized. Sometimes I join them, and it stops me from considering the future. So far, the "future" consists of free pop, lousy coffee, lots of bad television, and little fantasy circle jerks over the few good-looking nurses. Wes warned me early on that you would fall into this almost hypnotic daily ritual that anesthetized your brain and made you put one foot in front of the other (funny adage in the circumstances) without asking too many questions. Back then, I told him it would be a cold day in hell before I fell into a routine like that. Well, it is one motherfucking cold day in hell, and I didn't even see it coming.

CHAPTER TWENTY-SEVEN

DEPRESSION, AGAIN

MY PEOPLE AND MY FAMILY have not forgotten me; I get visitors. My sisters, parents, a friend or two. No one stays long. They try to cheer you up, pretend you're getting better, and then go on with their lives. Don't get me wrong, I like the visits, but I'm going through my own personal hell, and it turns out I'm not much of a sharer.

My life is the hospital and its people, mainly those who share my affliction. Carl is one of them. He should be leaving soon. He could have left one month ago, but he had nowhere to go. His buddies, the two I've seen, come about once every three weeks and load him up with enough pot to supply the whole seventh floor, which he does. I suspect his buddies—who look like they fell off the back end of a tractor and wouldn't get through the first page of a job application unless Dr. Seuss wrote it—have a grow operation somewhere out of town in their back forty and they make enough cash to keep their pickups filled with purple gas. They never stay long, and Carl just seems to tolerate them. I suspect they don't know how to deal with him in his new capacity as a Quad, and the feeling is mutual.

I can see why Carl is in no hurry to get out of the institution. Wes, Scott, and he are the best of friends, and in the hospital he is surrounded by like-minded people with the same physical impairment. Carl is essential in the hospital. He's the dope guy who gives you some encouragement in therapy because he's been there and done that. Young Dean thinks he's a great guy and hangs around him like a starry-eyed groupie. Carl pretty much has the run of the place. He's a big fish in a small pond, like the character played by George Segal in *King Rat*. You want something, Carl can quietly get it for you.

When we play the "What's Better Sweepstakes," Carl is the only one who considered having a brain injury a better option than being a Quadriplegic. I suspect Carl has no plans for the future and can't see past the next day. I envy him for his short-sightedness at times, but more often than not, I avoid him just in case his indifference is catchy.

It gives me pause to consider where I will find my role in the big scheme of all things necessary. I won't have all these fail-safe fallback positions once I clear hospital wavers. Right now, if my condom catheter comes unglued and I become a urine-soaked mess, there are always two or three nurses around to help me get cleaned up and back in my chair again. These nurses can't follow you home, and somehow I can't see my wife taking care of me without question or complaint. She doesn't mind coming to the hospital on her days off and spending time with me, and she is more than willing to take me places now, but things will change considerably as the restaurant gets up and running. However, her concerns are not my concerns, and all I know is that I won't stay in the hospital any longer than I have to. Fuck complacency, but I do know I'm not ready to leave quite yet.

Young Dean is probably in the same boat as me. He has maybe sixty days left on his sentence, then he'll be eligible for parole. They took away his plunger lance. His own personal self-destructive apparatus, or whatever you want to call it, and he seems in better spirits lately. After they took away his device, there was a time when he was inconsolable. I think that was because he derived some sense of importance from being "the only guy with enough guts to pull the plug when he's good and ready," as he was so fond of saying. Now he's at the institution's tender mercies, and the option of impaling himself is no longer open to him. His false bravado is dulled by time. Charlie, the counselor, still comes to see Young Dean, but he has given up on the rest of us. Wes curses him, Scott ignores him, and I give him my best "fuck you" steely-eyed look, and he steers clear. Vince the upright Para would talk to him for hours because Vince the upright Para would talk to a stump for an entire afternoon and come away happy. He is by far the most accepting of all of us and our circumstances.

Ten days after Charlie took away Young Dean's plunger lance, Young Dean took one last shot at ending his days on this Earth, and his ineptitude and embarrassment at failing in this endeavor kept him from trying anymore. It was a day when Althuna was in charge of the drug cart. Young Dean saw this as an opportunity and chose to follow the drug cart around from room to room, skulking in the background until Althuna left it unattended. Usually, two nurses were on the drug cart invariably, one of them was Arlene, and they were meticulous about where it was parked and how long it was left alone. Althuna had it all to herself on this day because the hospital was short-staffed, and it was a weekend. On weekends, the strokes and the no-brainers (head injuries) went home to see their families, leaving the Quads, the Paras, and the "Living Dead" to run the floor. Althuna left the cart alone mainly because she was trying to wrestle a cigarette out of Wes's hand, and he was putting up a pretty good fight. I could see Young Dean just outside the door at the drug cart, but I didn't think anything of it at the time.

After he smoked it to the nub, Wes finally gave up his cigarette, and Althuna finally shot me up with Demerol. By this time, Young Dean had scooped a handful of drugs out of three big bottles on the cart, and he scooted away before Althuna caught him.

He went back to his room, and twenty minutes later he came back to inform us that he was, once again, in control of his own destiny. He had put all his purloined pills into an old aspirin bottle he had in his drawer. I had to admit, he had a fair whack of medications, all in different fun colors.

"What did you get?" asked Wes, eyeing the pill bottle as Young Dean held it up.

"Orange ones mostly," said Young Dean, holding up his bottle and shaking it.

"What do the orange ones do?" I asked because the Demerol made the whole thing seem surreal, and it never occurred to me that Young Dean would actually take the pills.

"The orange ones are deadly," Young Dean explained in grave tones.

"How the hell do you know?" asked Wes.

"What other colors do you have?" I asked like I was on a street corner somewhere intending to purchase pills solely based on their color.

"Red ones and a handful of white ones," says Young Dean, like he knows what his stolen drugs represent.

"And I suppose the red ones are deadly too?" asked Wes, who couldn't keep the sarcasm out of his voice. I'm not sure why, but Young Dean went to great lengths to try to impress Wes.

"I suppose," says Young Dean, not sounding entirely sure.

"What difference does it make? You aren't going to take the fucking things anyway," I said, not wanting to make it sound like a challenge. I guess I was sick of Young Dean's pretentiousness and posturing. "If you're going to take the deadly red, white, and orange pills, then shut up and take them already," I finally said, hoping Young Dean would go away and let me get on with the business of being high on Demerol.

What happened next surprised both Wes and me as Young Dean grabbed up Wes's water jug, the one with the dents in it from smacking it on Thomas T. Thomas's head, and then he gulped the whole jug of water in his right hand while he poured handfuls of pills in his mouth with his left hand. He didn't stop until he had ingested the entire bottle of medications, and then Young Dean punctuated the proceedings by crashing down the water jug as if he'd just won a chugging contest at a college frat party. Wes and I just stared at him for the longest time until Wes finally broke the silence.

"You're fucking nuts," he said.

"Right fucking nuts," I echoed, "but I applaud your bravery."

Neither Wes nor myself even entertained the thought of pulling the ripcord at the time. We just sat there on that fine, lazy Saturday afternoon with the sun shining through the window and watched Young Dean. I don't know what we expected him to do, maybe spontaneously combust, turn green, or just keel over dead, but we patiently waited for his future to be decided.

"I don't feel anything," said Young Dean after what seemed like twenty minutes but was only about five.

"You don't look any different," said Wes stupidly.

"The pills probably take a half hour or so to work," I decided, with what seemed like flawless reasoning as if I was an expert on the over-ingestion of orange, red, and a handful of white pills and their effects. Wes had already lit up another smoke, and he was settling in for the long haul.

"What should I do?" asked Young Dean, as if he finally realized that he had probably taken an overdose of something and he wasn't quite sure how to react.

"The choices seem pretty fucking simple, stick your finger down your throat," suggested Wes, "Or just sit there so we can watch you die."

"That's too weird for me," I said as the Demerol kicked in. "Go back to your room to die, my little friend. You're freaking me out just sitting there."

"No way, fuck that, hang around," Wes pleaded. "We'll pull the ripcord if you start foaming at the mouth or speaking in tongues if that's what you want us to do?"

"I don't know," said Young Dean, looking small and confused. Finally, the gravity of his actions sank in, and the consequences weren't sitting well with him.

"Any last words?" asked Wes, like he was only too happy to witness Young Dean's final act, as usual deriving pleasure from someone else's misery.

So we sat there. All three of us bore witness—Wes in his bed, me in mine, and Young Dean in his chair between us—while the pills worked their way through Young Dean's system. We sat there for ten minutes, then ten more, and finally, even Young Dean got impatient.

"Nothing's happening," he complained. "My stomach hurts. That's about it."

"What kind of pills were they?" I asked. "And don't just say orange and red and white. I could see that. I'm just wondering what drugs they were."

"I don't know," admitted Young Dean. "The orange and red ones were in two big bottles, and the white ones were in a little tray. What do you think they were?"

"How the hell do I know? I take my drugs via syringe. Since you're the one that stole them, you'd think you might have taken a second to read the fucking labels," I said.

"I didn't have time."

"Well, whatever they were, they weren't as deadly as you thought they were," suggested Wes, sounding bored now that Young Dean was still alive and kicking. "Go back to your room and hang out. I'm taking a nap. At least I know the drugs I got were Morphine and Heparin, and that spells nap."

"My stomach really doesn't feel right," said Young Dean, still not convinced he wasn't going to die anytime soon.

"Oh, for Christ's sake," I finally said as I reached back and pulled the ripcord like I should've done when Young Dean scarfed the whole bottle down. But of course, this caused Young Dean some consternation, and he eventually pushed out of the room toward his own, and I was asleep before anyone ever answered the summons.

But four hours later, when I finally woke up, I was immediately worried about Young Dean. If any of the drugs he swallowed were of the fatal variety, they would have done their dirty work by now. I was greeted by Wes, wide-awake, smoking on a cigarette like nothing had happened, and I couldn't get the questions out fast enough.

"Where's Young Dean? What happened to him? I can't believe we just laid there and watched the guy take down a whole bottle of pills. Are we that fucking cold?" I said, reaching for the ripcord again to make sure someone had checked on Young Dean.

"Relax, Florence fucking Nightingale. Young Dean will survive to bitch another day."

"How can you be so sure?"

"Because nobody ever died from taking down a half bottle of Senecot and a half bottle of Colace. One is a stool softener and the other is a laxative times two. I think the white ones were Tylenol, but I can't be sure. So the only mad scramble was to get Young Dean on the commode chair before he fucking exploded like a big ass shit-bomb."

"No kidding. For fuck sake, I figured the kid for dead. I dreamed he was dead."

"Why would I kid about that? Our little fucked up friend Young Dean is about as useless as a goddamn two-wheel drive in a mud-pit when it comes down to killing himself."

"Holy shit, holy fucking shit," I managed to say, trying not to laugh. "That's funny," and then I'm laughing too hard to say much of anything else. Poor screwed-up Young Dean. He was more pathetic than tragic. I can't even talk for laughing, and Wes can't stop laughing either. Wes is laughing outright, and I'm not making a noise as my body shakes back and forth between wheezy sounds like *Dick Dastardly's Dog Muttley*. It's the best time I've had since I got here.

It's not as if Young Dean is without support. His mother, father, and sister are always around, encouraging him like his cheerleading squad. They accompany him to therapy. They fucking spoon-feed him. Young Dean is just young. Young and idealistic, and prone to be a little overdramatic. I fear these things will not serve him well on the road to recovery. I honestly believe a good dose of denial and cynicism is desperately needed if you intend to carry on a life outside the walls of the hospital.

Wes has cynicism in spades. He is a prick through and through, right to the core. He could watch a puppy drown and not bat an eyelid. There's just something missing in Wes. I still can't decide whether this was always the way with Wes, or if the accident and his fiancée took the last spark of humanity Wes was fanning into life and snuffed it out like a candle. I had learned that his childhood was less than idyllic, and that was obvious if you considered that not once did Wes receive a visitor other than his fiancée, and that didn't really count as a visit. It was more like a visitation.

I did learn that Wes's parents lived on a farm, and I could only surmise that they lived in the general area of Calgary. His immediate family life remained a mystery that was not easy to solve since Wes never volunteered information and wasn't especially good at answering questions. Fucking Paraplegic. Still, I envied his dexterity.

Wes was progressing at a satisfactory rate. Although he wasn't near as strong or as driven as Vince the upright Para, he made great strides in the transfer and push department. Wes got around the hospital real well, propelling his wheelchair at speeds I could only dream about. Everything about Wes's physical development was right on schedule, but mentally, holy shit, he needed work.

He refused to lift his ass off the chair and had three minor bedsores on his butt to prove it. Small ones, unlike the ones in the *Doctor Doom* worst-case scenario video where some bedsores were the size of Texas.

In itself, these small bedsores were not something to panic about since most Quads and Paras need a wake-up call on the positive aspects of good blood flow, but Wes just didn't seem to care. He also had a sore on his ankle and a perpetual bladder infection. Wes refused to shave lately, making him look like Keith Richards at a rehab clinic. His eyes were always red, and he kept his hair in a ponytail because then he wouldn't have to comb it. All these things, taken one at a time, were no big deal. But collectively, they added up to a general sense of apathy rarely seen in anyone except perhaps shipwrecked sailors after being in a lifeboat for six weeks without adequate food and water. They get that faraway, scary look in their eyes, and you don't want to be the fattest guy in the boat when the food runs out.

Wes just downright, out and out didn't care. Instead, he went about a typical day in a desultory, systematic way that let you know he was no longer overly interested in the curve balls life might throw him, and he did just enough to survive.

He was a man without a country; if he didn't personify the miserable prick stereotype, I would've felt almost sorry for him. But I had limited capabilities for that as I was too busy saving *myself* at this juncture in my life. Where I had reasons to keep going, Wes had none. I had a wife, and Wes didn't (nor did the immediate prospects look rosy). I had a restaurant to go to where I would attempt to notch out some valuable niche for myself (what that "niche" might be had yet to be determined), but Wes was unemployed and unemployable by all his accounts.

"What will you do once you get your walking papers?" I asked him one day. We had all developed this habit of calling our release from the hospital our walking papers because the irony wasn't lost. You think you can choose when to leave, but you just can't. The outside world was a scary place.

"Sweet fuck all," he replied. "I am throwing myself on the doorstep of Social Services, and they can fucking take care of me."

"Nice career choice."

"Yeah, well, fuck you too. I didn't ask to be a fucking Paraplegic. Nobody ever gave me anything, and now it's my turn."

"Turn for what?"

"To be a society leech. To live off the fat of the social system designed expressly for people like me." Unfortunately, Wes was having a bad day, even by Wes's standards.

"Have you been watching dis-empowerment videos or something? You're beginning to sound like Young Dean and his 'fuck the world' attitude."

"I'm just sick of trying, sick of listening to all that crap about how life will be full of slick little Kodak moments after I get out of this goddamn place."

"Well on the bright side, nobody can accuse you of being in denial."

"You got that straight."

"Well, now I'm curious," I said. "If someone like you, a Para, has no chance, where does that leave someone like me?"

"I'd bet on a snowstorm in the middle of the fucking desert before I bet on you making a go of that restaurant you and your wife are always carping about. Oh, sure, it'll start just fucking fine. They'll find some trivial little shit for you to do just so you ain't taking up space, but once the novelty wears off, they'll find a way to shove you out the door and replace you with somebody who can walk."

"Nice vote of confidence, dickhead."

"Don't mention it."

And there it was, that one-eighty switcheroo. That moment seems to perpetuate your hospital life. First, you're laughing your ass off thinking about Young Dean trying to kill himself by shitting himself to death, and then you are grimly reminded about your real-life situation. What could I do to help get a fledgling restaurant off the ground? Where did I fit in, and what could be my contribution? The doubts grow exponentially when doomsday Paras and suicide Quads surround you and poke little holes in your balloon. Confidence erodes pretty quickly in the hospital.

CHAPTER TWENTY-EIGHT

STEP THREE AGAIN: BARGAINING

DAY NINETY. THREE GODDAMN MONTHS, and Vince the upright Para is getting his walking papers. When he was the *almost* upright Para, he tried that much harder than anyone else in therapy, and the results speak for themselves.

This morning, Vince the upright Para crutched around the ward and said his goodbyes. He looks almost natural on his sticks. They clamp onto his thick forearms about halfway up, and he moves his legs in such a way that it imitates a walking motion, and you're left wondering where the crutches end and where the crippled Vince begins. He can even take about five steps using just his crutches. He's a show-off, but I love it. If anyone deserved a break, it was Vince. The happiest fucking guy on the seventh floor.

They brought a wheelchair for him earlier in the morning, but it would have been easier trying to drown a shark in a bathtub than to get Vince the upright Para to sit in it while they wheeled him out the door. He was determined that he was going out on his sticks, and nothing was going to stop him. We all went downstairs to watch him, the weirdest little cheering section on the planet. I think Young Dean cried a little.

Vince the upright Para will be missed. He is the least obtrusive person I have met in the hospital, and he offers nothing but encouragement and is always quick with a joke. He isn't contrary to anything, and I know he will be making return visits when he leaves. Because, in some strange way, he will miss us. We are both his audience and his measuring stick. Looking at our sad, sorry asses made him try that much harder. Vince is a survivor. He is annoyingly cheerful, but he would make it in the outside world, and he had Monique to help him.

Monique, the French nurse, had attached herself to Vince from the moment he was wheeled in, and she hadn't let go. She was by his side as he crutched from room to room in the morning, and finally, to great fanfare, when Vince crutched right out the front door. Monique, who looked even better in street clothes, went with him. For a brief moment, I envied him. Monique was also an optimist, a nurse that always offered positive feedback.

I asked Pam what was going on with that. It still seemed strange that Vince the upright Para could be attractive to Monique, who had her whole life ahead of her, and she didn't have to attach herself to a guy with no chance of ever walking properly again, let alone being a *whole* person.

"You're asking me?" asked Pam, looking incredulous.

"Yeah, because maybe you can explain it to me. Your husband is a Quadriplegic, and I need some insight here."

"I don't see my husband as a Quadriplegic," she said.

"So you're saying that Monique doesn't see Vince's crutches?"

"Yep."

"And you don't see your husband's wheelchair?"

"Precisely."

"Man, I don't get it. Where's the rub?"

"The person eventually eclipses the crutches, or in your case and my husband's case, the wheelchair."

"But the wheelchair defines you. It becomes who you are."

"You are so wrong, grasshopper. That's why Vince is leaving and you're not. He has essentially snatched the pebble from the proverbial hand, while you are still pushing a rope up the hill instead of pulling it."

"Huh?" I said, but she had turned away before I got anything resembling an explanation. Fucking Pam, who informed me that maybe I was done with denial and anger and was getting to bargaining, whatever that meant. Bargaining is the mysterious third step. Supposedly, you get to a point where you start to question your circumstances. The term "if only" is a big part of the process. "If only" my wife hadn't moved me. "If only" I had slept a couple of hours before getting behind the wheel. "If only" I had stopped at that last gas station before Lethbridge to stretch my legs and get a final cup of coffee. I'm still hoping, in the back of my mind (a long way back), that if I try harder in therapy, I will become more like Vince the upright Para, and the cure will come, some breakthrough excellent fucking remedy that will treat broken vertebrae and severed spinal cords. "If only" that would happen.

CHAPTER TWENTY-NINE

STEP TWO: ANGER, BIG TIME

I THINK IT IS DAY ninety-five or ninety-six, but I'm too drunk to remember if that was today or yesterday. I'm too drunk to do a lot of things.

I had been at the Keg for the last three hours, and I remember almost everything up to the fourth double tequila shooter with lime. From that point, things begin to get blurry around the edges.

We were celebrating something, but I can't remember what it was. Perhaps my un-triumphant return to the scene of the crime, the Keg, the fucking Keg, something that had happened a lifetime ago. Back when I was teeing up golf balls and firing them in the general direction of the condo complex across the road. Any excuse for a party worked for me. I was also celebrating my wife's second month of gainful employment at the Keg. It didn't matter. All that mattered at this moment was that I couldn't reach high enough to hit the button for the seventh floor.

I had been unceremoniously kicked to the curb two hours ago, or maybe it was three. The HandyDART (that beautiful rendition of a wheelchair taxi that I used back then) had a driver who waited long enough to make sure that his client had made it into the hospital. Once I had been buzzed in, I was no longer his responsibility. The lifers, or the hard-to-process people like me, had their own door, we avoided the Emergency Ward, and we got dropped off down a hill about a hundred yards away.

The notion of being buzzed into the hospital seemed ridiculous, as if anyone would want to go back to a hospital at around midnight unless they had to. More concerning to me: who was it that did the buzzing in and where were they now?

I had pushed, slowly to be sure, through the foyer to the elevators. There were three of them, but only one was open. I entered the elevator and had laboriously turned my chair in such a way as to give me access to the panel of buttons, only to find out that I couldn't lift my arm high enough to hit any one of the buttons. I could definitely not lift my arm high enough to hit the magical seventh-floor button. When pushed, that button would take me back up to my room and put me in the care of one of the overworked nurses that patrolled the floor from lights out until the morning shift changed at seven. I had come home late like this a couple of times before, but my dutiful wife had followed me upstairs and would have put me to bed if no one was available to assist her. When she was there, she had pushed the elevator buttons, so it never occurred to me that they might be out of my reach. Funny thing, I thought I was improving by leaps and bounds. I could hold my arms straight out and lift them to chest level. But now the whole Quad thing takes effect. My arm had now slammed into my nose, right eye (that'll leave a mark), and ear twice. My only hope was to somehow hit the magic seventh-floor button with my elbow.

Oh, the simple little things we take for granted. Try as I might—and I tried like a motherfucker—I couldn't maneuver my chair in such a way that the buttons were accessible. I went backward and forward twenty separate times to get closer. Finally, I had succeeded grandly at wedging myself into a corner where I could no longer go forward or backward, and my right arm was now pinned to the side of the elevator.

I sat like that for what seemed like hours, hoping against hope that whoever had buzzed me in was watching my progress—or non-progress, as the case may be. I wished hard that they would come from whatever small room they were in and rescue me. I waited, and I waited. I think I dozed off a couple of times, and at one point I tried yelling "HELLO" at the top of my lungs, but at no time did a person magically appear to push the special button and send me on my way.

Finally, after an interminable wait, the elevator door closed, and I let out an audible sigh of relief. The problem was that the elevator went down instead of up. When it stopped and the door opened, I found myself in the hospital's basement, the laundry room. The sound of tumbling dryers, the smell of laundry soap and detergent, and the humid warmth of the basement laundry room all came into the elevator. It wrapped itself around you like you were sticking your head in a dryer with wet clothes. It certainly led me to believe this was indeed the laundry room, but try as I might, I couldn't get myself unstuck so that I might explore my environs.

So here I am, way too late at night, waiting for someone to discover me in an elevator with my chair stuck in place, staring up at the seventh-floor button like it was the gold ring on the merry-go-round.

"A little help here," I yell to nobody in particular, and I imagine some demented person watching me on video, deriving some sick pleasure at my helplessness. Someone did buzz me in, after all.

"HEEELLLLLOOOOO," I yell again with the same ineffectiveness until my throat is parched, and I am convinced that I am the only person in the entire hospital.

It is an epiphany. I have seen the future. From this point forward, I will live my life like a drunk hobo on moonshine, worrying about getting stuck in elevators; claustrophobic, alone, and pathetic. In ten days, they will find me hungry, dehydrated, or very much dead, and I will have only myself to blame for trying to do too much all at once. A little dramatic, but I am drunk, so I fall asleep again. Contrary to what anyone might think, sleeping in a wheelchair is nigh impossible when the consequences of falling forward mean falling out of the chair and doing a header on the basement's concrete floor.

I finally snap just a little and start cursing and yelling in equal parts of unintelligible gibberish and frustrated half sentences. I finally free my hand, and I shake the chair back and forth and pound the metal walls of the elevator with my fists in a vain attempt to be noticed. I cannot remember a time when I felt so fucking helpless, like a baby trying to crawl out of its crib but the walls are too high.

Despite all my carrying on, nobody has noticed me, and when I finally calm down and achieve some Zen-like state of acceptance, I realize that patience will dominate my life in the future. This is because I am no longer in control. It is a harsh lesson to learn at two or three in the blessed a.m. in a hot, steamy laundry room of the hospital's basement.

But with the lesson comes a certain acceptance of one's fate, and I'm not even slightly disgusted with myself when I barf hot tequila shooter and undigested seafood onto my lap. It does not surprise me when my head starts to pound with an impending hangover. It's all just fate. It's all meant to be. I have hit the lowest point in my life, and I'm not even astounded, angry, or upset. I have been to hell (it sure smells like I imagine hell would smell), and I have to find a way back. This situational feeling can't be "acceptance," can it? The final step seems limp and unexciting. I expected fireworks, clowns doing cartwheels, or a fucking cake or something. The "What's Better Sweepstakes" has to include this scenario in the future.

Hours later, the elevator doors finally close again, and I go up and arrive at the third floor. Unfortunately, by this time I am slumped over. I have lost my compass. I am a Quadriplegic covered in tequila-seafood puke, too drunk to say where he belongs or how he got there.

Luckily, there are nurses on the third floor. Understanding, apologetic nurses, who are in no way responsible for what has befallen me, and I am relieved when they take me back to the seventh floor. I am cleaned up and put into bed, mumbling about the inequities of life. They had missed me, but they had assumed I went home with my wife and would eventually turn up.

They don't even try to wake me up in the morning. It is the first time I have missed therapy in six weeks.

CHAPTER THIRTY

MORE DENIAL, ANGER, AND BARGAINING

THEY HAVE A MEETING ABOUT me that afternoon, and my attendance is required. My feeling is that the nursing staff is worried about me. I have hit the imaginary wall. It will have been over three months since my involuntary admission into the hospital, and three months is the seemingly arbitrary, random number of days they gave me to show a marked improvement. "We'll know more in three months" was the statement that I (and especially my wife) attached ourselves to and held onto for hope. I hugged it like a mother hugs a newborn.

Three months is pretty much up, and there's very little chance that I will get any better. This is my new reality. Finally, I have gotten back all the feeling and the movement that my research and intuition told me I would get back. So, I am grudgingly making my way to the ticker-tape parade that spells acceptance.

I have officially (almost) maxed out improvement-wise, and I am now paralyzed forever from the shoulders down. One inch above the nipples on the chest and one inch above the shoulder blades on the backside, reverse side, or any other fucking side.

My biceps work; my triceps don't. My wrists flex upward, palms down, and they don't curl one iota if my hands are palms up. I have deltoids and shoulder muscles, trapezoid muscles, and the top of my forearms. I can feel the texture of stuff I touch with the tips of my thumbs, and I have some residual feeling in my index fingers.

That is it, and that is all there is going to be. So why the meeting? And why would they make me and my wife wait in the hall until they call us? I feel like I'm back in third grade and outside the principal's office. Of course, I sat outside a principal's office a lot, but it just got old after third grade, so get on with the fucking punishment already.

"It must have been pretty scary sitting in the elevator in the basement last night," my wife says again, for the third or fourth time. She is nervous that we've done something wrong and they will take away our membership privileges or something.

"Not scary, just lonely, and . . . helpless, right fucking helpless. It brought the disability home with a bang. I feel I'm going to be in that situation more than once, and that is ultimately scary . . . But, ah, fuck it, I'm such a drama queen," I say in response.

"You're not going to be alone," she says.

"Define alone, 'cause it sure felt alone to me," I say. After I say it, I realize I'm such a dick. I wish the principal would come out and get this fucking charade over with and give me the proverbial strap, an anachronism for sure. What the fuck do kids get nowadays? It is probably a firm "talking to" in a meeting with parents and a counselor present, so they are not scarred for life. Give me the strap or detention, tell me they expected more from me, and they're all damn disappointed. I've heard that shit a thousand times. Just let me get my hungover ass back to bed. I can still smell the puke in my lap from the night before.

"I'll always be there. I'm not going anywhere," my wife says, just adding extra words to my already filled-up head.

"That's not what I'm afraid of," I say, and I know she is confused, but I don't feel like explaining how a whole room can be filled with people and you can still be alone. Thank Christ I'm saved an explanation when Nurse Pam finally comes out, and we're ushered into the small conference room. I nod at Monique and Nurse Chalmers, making a surprise guest appearance. *Doctor Doom* and the Charge Nurse are present. The Charge Nurse who pushes paper and people and can't distinguish one from the other, I think her name is Hilda. I wonder where Althuna is since she seems to be involved in my care and feeding, but I'm guessing her English skills are not quite up to snuff, so she probably wasn't invited. And where is Arlene, who wiped Keg seafood and tequila puke off me this morning? *Doctor Doom* claps his hands and clears his throat.

"Randy, I was alarmed to hear about your little incident last night, and I think it's time we addressed what we expect of you from here on out." *Doctor Doom* had chucked the whole bedside manner thing.

"If you tell me right now how it's an 'exciting time to be a Quad,' I might manage to throw something heavy, sharp, and hopefully lethal at you," I say.

"No, I'm not going to say that at all. I just want to reiterate our mission at this time."

"Your mission? *Your* fucking mission?" I don't even realize I'm close to yelling, but I can see it has the desired effect.

"Yes, you seem to think this is some kind of hotel set up for your convenience where you can come and go as you please, and that isn't what we're here for. We're here to get you acclimated to your condition so you might function better when it's time for you to get out of the hospital."

"So you want me to stay away from the outside until you have acclimatized me to the outside?"

"Precisely . . . well, not exactly. We are here to help you improve your condition, and then when we think you're ready to be released, you can go home and later come and go as you please, but not with the auspices of the hospital at your disposal."

"I will tell you right now that there won't be any 'come and go as I please' because I won't be coming back once I'm released."

"That is our goal, yes," he reiterates, back on familiar ground.

"So . . . I should stay here until I'm well enough to come and go as I please, and then I can go? And you can shove your auspices. I won't need them."

"Uh, yes. I think that's what I'm getting at."

"Ooookay," I say real slowly, like I'm genuinely not understanding any of this, and I try a thumbs up, but it's beyond my limited capacity. It looks like I'm extending my fist to be bumped.

"Good," says *Doctor Doom* triumphantly. "I thought that would be a struggle. I'm glad you understand. I guess that's all we had to get across to you, and I'm sure you have some therapy sessions to attend unless you've already missed them, so I'll make my rounds. Hilda can answer any questions you have," he states while he's packing up his binder and his charts, and he's out the door before anyone else has had a chance to speak.

After he's vacated the room, I look at Nurse Pam because she's grinning and seems to sense my absolute confusion. Nurse Hilda, the aforementioned sometimes nurse slash paper pusher, has never been too forthcoming with information. Hence, she isn't my go-to person on this anyway. However, she has told me her name numerous times upon my request, and I forget it two minutes after she tells me because she has attributed little to my general well-being.

"What the hell just happened here?" I ask Pam.

"He doesn't want you drinking, and he especially doesn't want you coming back to the hospital late, helpless, and drunk."

"That's it? Why didn't he just say so?"

"He did in his own way. You know it's been about three months since you've been with us, don't you?"

"Yeah, right, like I'm going to lose track of that. You make it sound like a choice."

"Since it's been three months, your prognosis changed somewhat."

"You're going to tell me I've peaked, aren't you?"

"Not necessarily," says Pam, shaking her head. "You will improve tremendously and adapt accordingly to what you've already got back. You're not likely . . . no, you're very *unlikely* to get any more feeling or movement back, although some feelings return even after four years, although I'm more inclined to think that you just get better at working with what you already have. The bottom line is that we will work with the returned sensations. It will probably be another couple of months before we cut you loose, but during that time, try to take the therapy seriously, lay off the late-night binging, and especially try to stay away from elevators." She grins because I know she finds that whole situation funny.

She then turns around and looks directly at my wife. "Eventually you'll have to look at making your living quarters more accessible, if that hasn't already happened, and you and Randy will have to talk about getting care outside the hospital once he's released." This last bit is solely for my wife's benefit.

"I can take care of him," she says defensively, more by rote than anything else. She looks like she just missed being hit by an avalanche and is still shocked that she's the lone survivor. The true impact of what has been happening around her is just beginning to sink in. In reality, the simple phrase, "Taking care of me," sounds ominous to both her and me.

"I think you probably can," says Pam patiently. "But I wouldn't advise it, and I have some experience in that regard."

"So what should we do?" my wife asks, looking defeated for the first time, slumping like a tire tube without air.

"Don't panic. That's number one. We're not going to throw Randy out in the parking lot, although that was mentioned as an option earlier," and I noticed she flicked a glance at Hilda. "So you have plenty of time, and I can help you a lot in some areas. If you feel like it, maybe you and Randy can come over for dinner one night to our place, and you might get some ideas." Hilda sniffs like there has been some discussion about this earlier, and she disapproves. She seems to disapprove a lot.

"Sure," my wife says, more than happy to find an ally after feeling like she's been bushwhacked. I wonder again if it had genuinely occurred to her that my "condition," as *Doctor Doom* called it, was not going to improve dramatically. Is it just sinking in? Three months go by pretty quickly in her mind. It feels like three years in mine.

"How about seven tonight, and we'll have him back before curfew?" Pam asks, and my wife agrees before I am ever consulted or could protest. Going to Pam's seems wrong somehow, like it violates the patient-nurse relationship, and besides, I am in the middle of a deadly hangover.

After that, the meeting breaks up, and my wife pushes me back to my room. We're alone because Wes is up on the eighth floor with Scott discussing the various ways two guys in wheelchairs can run successful marijuana grow operations in a double-wide trailer, and they won't be back for hours.

"You don't mind going to Pam's, do you?" my wife asks after I've been helped back into bed. I'm still exhausted from the adventure I had last night and fully intended to sleep the rest of the afternoon or my life away, with my close friend Demerol.

"A little. I don't know if I feel comfortable meeting some other Quad on the outside in a home setting, or I keep thinking this is a bad dream, and the more involved I get, the harder it will be to wake up. I guess it just feels like everything is happening too fast."

"What do you mean?"

"It's like the first couple of months went by real slow, probably because I didn't know what to expect, and everything was new and a struggle. Now that I know this is how much I'm getting back, time has sped up considerably. I feel like I'm crashing back to Earth without a parachute."

"Didn't you hear what Pam said? You can still get some return after four years." My wife looks hopeful.

"I think they're talking about something as small as a twitch in your little finger or a two percent improvement in your triceps, which amounts to sweet fuck all in the end."

"Quit being so negative."

"Yeah, easy for you to say. Fuck you." That last bit was wholly unnecessary.

"Nothing about this is easy for me either, you know."

"Right, you don't have to sit like a crow on a wire over a toilet with five or six other people separated by a partition every other morning, hoping you crap to such a degree that you won't do it later in your pants when you're not expecting it. You aren't spoon-fed because you can't hold a fucking utensil. You don't have to sit in a fucking elevator with puke on your shoes, hoping somebody finds you before breakfast so you can eat another delicious bowl of goddamn Red River Cereal with powdered milk and cold-as-ice fucking toast."

"Well, fuck you too. It's not like I fell asleep and crashed the truck," my wife says vehemently, and it takes the wind out of my sails.

"Yeah, yeah, I hear you. It's such a giant pain in the ass, and I keep thinking everything will be back to the way it was if I'm patient. Like I'm getting some fucking test, and it's supposed to make me a better person, only I can't see the end."

"Oh great, anger and denial and bargaining. Pam and Monique told me about this. The five steps of recovery."

"Go away. I want to sleep. Besides, you've got to come back so we can play Quads on parade at Pam's tonight. You were planning on going with me, I hope."

"I'll go," she says, and I can tell she's as excited about this dinner as I am, so why did she readily accept? Safety in numbers, sharing responsibility? I sure as hell hope she doesn't think that because I'm a Quad, all of our new circle of friends must have this affliction in common.

"Bring beer and wine, " I say as she's leaving. "Even with a curfew, I can still be a lush. The curfew alone inspires me to greater heights of lushdom."

She gives me a look that says "bite me" better than words could, and she's gone, leaving me with my little pathetic self. It's not the first time I wondered where that plunger lance we built for Young Dean is hiding.

CHAPTER THIRTY-ONE

STEP FOUR: DEPRESSION, NASTY DEPRESSION

MY WIFE IS ALMOST RIGHT on time. That, in itself, is rather amazing because late is a way of life for her lately, and being severely delinquent is not uncommon. Secretly, I was hoping she would have second thoughts and not show up at all. But instead, I've been up and waiting for the last twenty minutes, thinking and worrying about how I'm going to get to Pam's without ending up in a parking lot somewhere with two women who might or might not be able to pick me up.

I already hate loading myself into the car. Although I would be the first to admit I do very little of the work myself, it is still not getting any more manageable, and I'm wondering if it ever will. Pam has volunteered to drive on this little outing. She gets off work, and we head to the parking lot.

"I phoned Peter ahead of time so he knows we're coming, and advised him of the dinner plans," she says, and I'm wondering what possible difference this could make to Peter. "This way, he can crank up the oven, start the roast, and throw on a couple of baked potatoes. I hope that's okay with you guys?"

"Yeah, that's fine," says my wife.

"Whoa," I say, not about to let this go by unchallenged. I had imagined that husband Peter, coincidentally named after my I.V. pole, had broken his neck in the C5 region much as I did. I assumed he would be hanging around home, stored in a closet somewhere like the vacuum cleaner or the dust mop, or at best be lying around in bed until Pam got him out and made him wheelchair ready. To hear that he is capable and willing to "crank up" the oven without help leaves me feeling slightly inadequate. I have thought ahead as far as my limited imagination will allow me to, and I cannot see a future where my wife will call from work and ask me to "crank up" anything, let alone the oven, and start a roast or bake a potato.

"Aren't you afraid he's going to burn the house down or light himself on fire?" I ask, knowing this is a teaching moment and I should pay attention, something I never did in school.

"No, he cooks quite a bit. Simple stuff, really, nothing complicated. He's the shits at slicing up vegetables, so I always buy pre-made salads and stuff, but he can start the barbecue or put something in the oven."

"Talented little bugger, isn't he . . . I suppose I'm about to get a lesson on what I can do after leaving the hospital. Is that part of what this little road trip is about?"

"Make of it what you will. Keep an open mind and maybe you'll pick up a few tips. It's not difficult to compare the two of you. It's just a way of getting some perspective, maybe for you both."

I feel like telling her where she can shove her perspective, but my wife seems eager and happier than she was earlier this afternoon. I wonder once more about that three-month cut-off where all hope for recovery is suspended, and I question the geniuses who came up with this subjective period that dashes hopes on the rocks, much like you'd break an egg with a mallet. My head hurts like hell, but I mentally make a note not to let cynicism rule the night ahead and do just what the nurse ordered, and that would be to keep an open mind—oh, and have someone wash my shoes. They still smell like last night's dinner.

The wheelchair-accessible van that Pam owns is a delightful surprise. It flat out kicks ass. It is so smooth and practical that I can't think of a reason why I would ever want to be transferred into a car seat again. The door opens up automatically, and a slick little ramp descends on a perfect downward slope and comes to rest on level ground. Of course, it's child's play to roll onto the ramp, and before you can say Thomas T. Thomas three times, I am settled in and belted down. I try not to appear too impressed. However, what I've been through in the transfer department, what with being picked up off the ground in four separate yet equally unnerving incidents in four different parking lots, this van seems more like a magic carpet than just a simple motor vehicle. Score one for Pam and Peter.

They don't live far from the hospital, so a mere twenty minutes later I'm rolling up to the door of a three-bedroom condo built entirely on the ground level. Pam opens the door with a large flat metal key that wouldn't look out of place hitting ping-pong balls, and she explains how easy it makes it for Peter to get in and out and lock the door behind him. Peter, it seems, does everything but fly planes and rock climb, and I'm not sure I want to meet him anymore. This is not a comparison. Instead, it's a rebuke of my usefulness.

Peter is at the front door waiting for us when we enter. I insist on pushing pathetically in my pre-sixties wheelchair with hard rubber wheels. This fucking thing was invented before pneumatics were a thing. The wheels will never pop and leave you stranded. I go at a speed that wouldn't win me a newborn crawling contest, but the big thing is that I, and I alone, propel the wheelchair forward. Hooray for fucking me.

"Howdy," says Peter. Howdy is a relatively common greeting in Calgary, and he looks like he wears his howdy with noticeable aplomb. He's dressed in jeans and a nifty cowboy shirt with snappy pearl buttons, and on his head is a large cowboy hat, about as gaudy and conspicuous as colorful rainbow sprinkles on vanilla ice cream. I've never been a good judge of volume when it comes to cowboy hats, but I'm betting this one is one of those ten-gallon jobs if it's an ounce.

"Howdy," I return with enthusiasm, which prompts a quick elbow from my wife, who knows I'm not the howdy type. "You must be Peter?"

"You betcha," and with that, he holds his limp hand out for me to shake, and I'm at a loss about what I'm supposed to do next. One of the things Quads do not do well, among other things, is shake fucking hands. Shaking hands with another Quad is damn near impossible. I touch my chin and give him a little salute, leaving his hand right where it is. I'm not about to start the night out playing fumble fingers with another Quad I don't even know. He doesn't push the exchange and instead backs up his electric wheelchair and moves out of the way, allowing me to make my way into the house. It has hardwood floors, so a bit of push goes a long way. Hardwood is definitely the way to go. There's nothing like a carpet for sucking up pure pushing energy. It is the equivalent of running in thick mud with ankle weights. Note to me; find out how expensive hardwood is and put it everywhere.

Peter backs up and quickly spins around in the foyer. He operates the electric chair like it is a part of him. He doesn't even look where he's going. I sit in awe.

He's not a big guy. Point of fact, he's relatively small, dwarfed by the chair he sits in. He has a pot-belly, and his back has a decided curve in it. His head sits forward on his bony shoulders like he's trying to see the tops of his shoes. He appears to be about five and a half feet tall, and his toes point inwards, causing his legs to bow slightly. His long black hair is tied back in a ponytail fashion, and he's sporting a pencil-thin mustache, which gives him a Mexican heritage appearance. I can't help thinking of the *Jimmy Buffett* song "Pencil Thin Mustache." He has a big inviting smile and perfect white teeth accentuating his tan. His hat, after further inspection, looks way too big for his head. It is a ten-gallon hat on a five-gallon head. He spins around in another quick one-eighty, and I am surprised as fuck that his hat stays on. It must be velcroed to his head.

"Want a beer?" he asks, and before I can say yes or no—my answer seems pretty damn evident since I've got twenty-four cold ones on my lap—my wife peremptorily removes the cold ones, making me feel naked. I watch Peter as he zips into the kitchen, opens the fridge, reaches in, and grabs me a cold one. After which, he shoots forward in his chair to give it to me. I'm cringing, thinking he plans to run me and my little pushchair right back out the door, but he stops dead right in front of me, and my wife takes the beer out of his hands as he does another half spin and heads back toward what must be the main living area of the house. It's like following the progress of a water bug as it skips around on a clear pond. He never stays still for more than a second. I think he's showing off.

"Come on in," he says as Pam takes off her shoes, and I take a deep breath and ready myself for another excruciatingly slow push. I suffer another acute pang of electric wheelchair envy. I give my wife the cold beer and a-pushing we shall go.

The living room is vast, with all hardwood floors and an open area that makes the one comfortable couch look conspicuously out of place. There are no rugs and no coffee table, no impediments whatsoever. It is a living room designed for somebody who doesn't want a whole lot of roadblocks as he's going from point A to point B. It was the first time I realized furniture would no longer have meaning or importance in my life. So what do I care for recliners and ottomans (fuck you recliners, I used to love you) when I'm stuck sitting in the chair that brought me here?

"Want to check out the rest of the place?" asks Peter, addressing me instead of my wife. I am obviously the focus of this experiment, and I mutter my answer.

"In for a penny, in for a pound," I say, and slowly (painfully slowly) I follow him through the living room and down a wide hallway, where I can park myself in the middle, reach out, and barely touch both walls. He enters the first room to the left, and I laboriously follow behind him, still grumbling about pennies and pounds.

"The bathroom," he announces as he does a half-hearted hand swoop with ill-concealed pride as if we had just entered a shrine to all that is important in this life. It is much too much for me, and I start laughing.

"What's so funny?" he asks, looking hurt or confused. I don't know which.

"You don't find it funny that I don't even know you, and you can't wait to show me the bathroom of your house, which you take great pride and delight in displaying? You don't find that just a little weird?"

"Oh, right," he says, slightly smacking himself in the forehead, making his hat jump around. Okay, so it's not velcroed. "You're a rookie," he continues. "It probably hasn't even occurred to you that this will be one of the most important rooms in your house or apartment. Give it time, and you'll clue right in. When you get stuck in a bathroom between the toilet and the tub, or you find yourself unable to turn around or even turn on the taps, then you'll understand."

"I can't wait," I say, trying hard not to sound sarcastic as I take in my surroundings. It is probably the most enormous bathroom I've ever been in. You could park a fucking Buick in it and still open the doors. He has what looks like a mini hot tub in one corner and what appears to be a small crane with a sling-type device hooked up beside it. The counters are extended outwards from the wall, and you can roll right under the sinks, which have touch-control faucets where you lift or push down to control temperature and flow. I can't resist rolling under the counter to try them out. I have now caught the spirit of the tour.

"The Hoyer lift is controlled by a little box that hangs up on the wall. You hook the straps under your thighs and your ass, and you can lower right into the tub," he explains, pointing to various pieces of the sling-like device. I'm not listening as I turn the tap on and off, adjusting the temperature as if I had just discovered water for the first time, but I try to look suitably impressed, which allows him to continue to espouse the virtues of the Hoyer lift. I finally stop playing with the taps for the moment, and I take in the rest of the bathroom at a glance, but before I can comment, he's beckoning me out the door and heading down the hall again. I follow dutifully behind him, maintaining a steady pace of about a tenth of a mile an hour. I notice my wife is not keeping up with the tour. Her tour guide is slower than mine. I can hear the whir of machinery in the bathroom, and I can listen to Pam explaining the fine points of the thing Pete, the curator and guide, had called a Hoyer lift. I gamely continue without her, following the water bug. He skips down the hall into a room on the right. Fuck me, does my head hurt. I decide it's best to drink myself out of this hangover. I want my beer and maybe another ten after that.

"The master bedroom," he announces. He's big on promoting shit, as if this "master bedroom" wasn't obvious. "That's the waterbed. It saves me from moving around so much and stops me from getting bedsores." This elicits another chuckle from me. I once again shake my head. The surreal weirdness of the personal comments coming from this guy is freaking me out. I haven't even had a chance to hang up my coat or get my bearings. Peter must be so used to his life being an open book that this does not seem strange to him. I decide to go with the flow.

"Who puts you to bed?" I ask before I think this question might be personal, but there is no such thing. He picks up the ball and runs with it.

"Watch this," he says and spins close to the bedside like a race car driver pulling into the pits. He flips his little legs up on the bed, and lickety-split, he transfers his ass over onto the bed. From there, he bends forward and moves closer to the middle, at which point he flops back on the pillows like a man hell-bent on taking a nap. He lies there for a second, causing me to wonder if that is what he intends to do, until I notice him fumbling with a rope ladder attached to the end of the bed. After gaining purchase on one of the material rungs—like a rope ladder with rungs every ten inches—he brings himself up on one elbow and then sits up. I assume he's trying to show me how easy it is for him to get around on his own without aid, but again, before the question period can begin, he transfers back into his chair with one big heave. His little legs fall off the bed only to be directed to their proper places in the foot pedals. It's quite a performance, one undoubtedly worthy of praise.

"Your pants are all twisted up," I observe. The guy has just performed a trick comparable to making a hippopotamus disappear into a phone booth, and I remark about how twisted his pants are—goddamn afternoon hangover.

"Yeah, it's something I'm working on. It's worse in the morning. Sometimes it takes me three-quarters of an hour to dress."

"Three-quarters of an hour," I say, surprised, with my mouth open. The time spent on this enterprise seems inordinately ridiculous to me.

"Depends whether I'm having a routine. I need help with my routine," Peter admits rather sheepishly.

"So somebody helps you with the suppository commode chair thing, yet you insist on dressing yourself?"

"Sure, it makes me feel independent."

"Independent," I say, incredulous, knowing that he doesn't see the irony in this.

"You betcha. Velcro straps do up my shoes, and I've got little loops in the waist of my pants so I can get them pulled up. It's taken me years to get to a point where I can get up by myself every morning."

"And this is a point of pride?" I ask. I'm getting sick of this Quad version of what amounts to little more than a long-dong competition.

"You betcha," he says because he does not recognize sarcasm.

"Man, you've got way too much time on your hands. I don't get it. You struggle for an hour with something someone else can do in five minutes. This is a gross misuse of valuable time. It's like using a tin can and a string long after the invention of the fucking telephone. It's like opening a can with a rock or cooking food over a fucking campfire. Are you nuts?"

"What are you two plotting?" asks Pam as she comes into the room with my wife in tow.

"I'm teaching this guy how to be a productive Quad," I tell her. "He's just not using the resources available to him. Now, where did my wife put that beer?" I go to push back toward the kitchen, and my hands slip off the wheels. I almost fall forward over my legs. My wife quickly shoves me back up, and she takes over the pushing from there. I can't resist a big shit-eating grin aimed in Peter's general direction while I let others do unto me as I cannot do unto myself. However, I get a slight feeling of independence when I push my chair unassisted. Still, Peter must realize that time management is a massive thing to me, although this is not the time or place to mention it.

I drink eight beers (I notice because I am the only one drinking), and I have a delicious roast, which Peter insists on cutting up himself. He has a wicked-looking, accident-waiting-to-happen electric knife, and I make another mental note to get me one of those. In the end, we sit back in the living room and have a coffee. I speak again about letting people do things for you.

"Why take an hour out of your day doing the mundane crap that would take someone else ten minutes?" I ask in a reasonable tone. I haven't made any converts on this point, and I find this very irritating. I realize that quality of life means being independent in every way possible, but not at the expense of valuable time spent doing something that doesn't improve your feelings of well-being. There is time well spent and time frivolously wasted; you've got to know the difference.

"When I dress myself," says Peter, in an equally reasonable tone, "I feel better about my place in the world. It is as if God has ordained that I must persevere and overcome the little obstacles 'He' puts before me so that I might be a better person."

"Huh?" In what might be construed as confusion, more disbelief than confusion is evident if someone listens closely. I get the same feeling in the pit of my stomach that comes when the sports interviewer asks an outstanding athlete how he managed to hit five home runs in one game or knock out Mike Tyson. I just don't get it when the first thing they do is go into a euphoric harangue thanking God for everything they have achieved. I want to reach through the television and smack them upside the head. Like God had anything to do with it. Maybe that's why hockey is my favorite spectator sport. It's all about the game. It's rare that someone gives God any credit.

"So, what you're talking about here . . ." I say slowly, stopping theatrically, like I'm mulling this over when I'm looking to reach across the table and do a knuckle dance on his smiling beatific face. My wife knows this and tries to say something soothing, but I say the same thing only louder before she can interrupt. "So, what you are saying . . . is that doing something counterproductive, and I might mention, time consumingly moronic, makes you feel closer to God. He's a tough sell, this God guy you keep mentioning."

"Wag," says my wife, knowing that I'm working myself into a frothy, full-blown rant. "Maybe you should save this for some other time."

"No, let him say what he wants," says Pam, and I'm about four beers too late to care what Pam thinks anyway, and I'm about to nail my point home in true drunken rant fashion when Peter speaks again. My hangover is a distant memory.

"God has a plan . . ." mulls Peter. "He has a plan for all of us."

"And what might that fucking plan be? Does 'He' plan to let us screw up the entire goddamn planet to the point of extinction and destruction until 'He' finally deals himself back into the game? It's so arrogant and self-important to think that in all this vast universe, we are God's chosen fucking people, or does every newly-discovered solar system get its own God or version thereof? You have to fall off more than one vegetable cart to think Adam and Eve and the garden of fucking Eden ever existed. Like they wouldn't have gotten their defenseless naked little asses chewed off by the first Tyrannosaurus rex they encountered, unless dinosaurs never truly existed. And Noah? Give me a break. That would make the entire animal kingdom, and us included, founded on incestuous relationships. Didn't Charles Darwin teach you anything, or did you close your eyes and wish you were back in Kansas during grade school? Let's just forget science. Oh, the hell with it. Sorry, partner, I'm just not a convert. Religion can justify anything and explain away ignorance faster and slicker than a Nolan Ryan fastball, and it produces more misguided energy than a teenager with his first hard-on." Luckily, it's about then that I run out of gas and lengthy metaphors.

"You have the right to your opinion," says Peter, and it occurs to me that he's the first God-fearing person that ever told me that. It's enough to make me pause for a breath, but before I can get started again, my wife cuts me off with a look that could bend forged steel and kill the aforementioned dinosaurs.

"I think it's time for us to go," she says. "Thanks for having us over. We appreciate this," and she's pushing me toward the door before I can wind myself up again.

She needn't have worried. I'm super tired. I think the whole day caught up to me in one big rush, and I can't wait to get loaded up and roll on back to the safe confines of the hospital. I say my goodbyes, and we're in the van lickety-split. I think again about how I can't wait to get me one of these babies.

Pam semi-apologizes, but her contriteness is an act. I can't shake the feeling that, in some way, what occurred between Peter and I was scripted, and since I have no desire to go into motives, I accept the apology and carry on. But unfortunately, my wife is not so eager to let it rest this time.

"Was Peter always religious?" she asks.

"No, not always," says Pam, sighing heavily. "He got into it big time in the last six months. I must admit that, at first, I didn't mind because he was getting so depressed for a while that I thought anything that took his mind off the business of being depressed couldn't be a bad thing. But now I'm not so sure. He keeps sermonizing to the point where I want to shake him, and he doesn't have time anymore for anything else except the church he goes to and the people who belong to it."

"So, what's the worst that could happen?" I ask. "His head hasn't been turning in circles, and he doesn't speak in tongues, so why worry? I wouldn't panic unless he offers you a glass of Kool-Aid or starts getting overly excited about the next comet coming through. Religion preys on the weak and impressionable. People that need crutches mentally and physically. I shouldn't be so goddamned judgmental. Whatever gets you through the night, man, unless this wheelchair shit gets a whole hell of a lot easier, what can it hurt?"

"Have you considered a religion?"

"Not bloody likely. Haven't you been listening? I'm too arrogant and self-important for that load of hypocrisy," I say before I realize I'm slagging Peter by saying this.

Pam says little else on the way back to the hospital. I can't help but get excited all over again about the nifty wheelchair ramp as it plunks me back on the ground. It's such a simple thing to get excited about, but it'll never get old. I could watch this thing for days. After she unloads the both of us and says a hurried goodbye, she takes off without another mention about the night we just spent together.

"Kind of strange, don't you think?" my wife remarks. "I thought we were going over there to be reassured, but I got the impression it was the other way around."

"Me too," I say. "Something is not quite right in that house. I don't want to suggest that living with a Quad is easy; it ain't Disneyland, but maybe that's part of the problem. We truly don't know what we're up against yet."

"We won't have a problem," my wife assures me, and I readily agree because what else can I do? Scare her by telling her what a nightmare it's going to be living with someone who requires care constantly?

But the point is hammered home as she pushes another button I can't quite reach (fucking buttons) and speaks to the hospital's version of a doorman that allows us to enter the hospital. After this, the doorman goes back to sleep, reads his book, or sticks his thumb back up his ass, if the situation I found myself in this morning is an example. I'm just glad my wife follows me up to the seventh floor, pushing all the right buttons in the elevator and ensuring that a nurse is willing to put me to bed. I am happy not to repeat the laundry room experience.

Arlene, efficient as always, deposits me in my bed, and she bustles out as soon as I'm settled. The hospital is quiet tonight. I can hear Wes breathing imperceptibly about ten feet away, knowing he's fast asleep because he hasn't made a snide or questionable comment. My wife hangs around for a while, but she is thoughtful and preoccupied. I'm guessing she's rethinking her earlier critique about how "easy" it will be to live with a Quad.

"We're going to have to do a lot of renovations to our apartment," I say, guessing that this is indeed the reason for part of her dismay. "There isn't an elevator in the building, and it bears mentioning that we live on the third floor."

"Yes, and I'm already doing something about it. We can have the first apartment available on the bottom floor, and the management is putting in a ramp by the side door. I was going to surprise you with this information a little way down the road, but it seems they're in a hurry to get you out of here."

"You're way ahead of me. Have the contractors started building the restaurant yet?" Construction was supposed to start sometime last month, if memory serves, but I haven't inquired about it. I've been avoiding talk of the restaurant and the huge undertaking of starting and running it while I'm adjusting to life in a wheelchair. Finally, she comes back, sits on the bed corner, and sighs heavily. I can tell we are about to discuss the restaurant at some length.

"Have you thought about what you want to do in the restaurant?" she asks.

"Strange question. I assumed I would still be the kitchen manager. I just won't manage by example. Instead, I will delegate and point and yell obscenities when necessary and endeavor not to cut any of my fingers off."

"Be serious. How about keeping the books?" my wife asks.

"How about it?" I ask back.

"Could you see yourself doing something along those lines?"

"Um, let me see. I hate bookkeeping, and I don't know squat about computers. I suck at math, and I'm sure as hell not going to keep the books and let someone else manage the kitchen. So that should let you know how jazzed up I am about bookkeeping."

"You could learn."

"Why don't we cross that bridge when we get to it?" I say. "We have more to worry about than who keeps the books. At some point, long before bookkeeping becomes a priority, we'll have to hire staff, set up suppliers, get all the kitchen stuff installed, choose fucking carpet colors, and take care of about a gazillion other little details."

"The restaurant will be done in four months, maybe five. Will you be out of the hospital by then?" she asks hopefully.

"The powers that be, the ones making all the decisions in this hospital, seem to think so."

"Did you check out all the neat stuff Peter had? That Hoyer lift would come in handy."

"You would have to build a house around a Hoyer lift. One of those things would take up your entire bathroom," I say pointedly. This is a lot of stuff to digest already.

"Yeah, yeah, I know. We'll cross that bridge when we come to it. I'm just getting a little worried about how hard it will be when you get out of the hospital. We have to hire a nurse or a care-aide or something."

"We'll manage. How tough can it be?" I was maintaining a brave front. I had a lot of questions about just how I was going to exist outside the hospital, but I couldn't answer these questions until I graduated from the hospital. It was going to be one long, long bridge by the time we crossed it.

CHAPTER THIRTY-TWO

STEP ONE: DENIAL ONE MORE TIME, AND STEP FOUR: DEPRESSION

PAM IS THERE THE FOLLOWING day when I wake up. She seems subdued as she dresses Wes, as she doesn't even address the cigarette he's smoking. Wes doesn't require as much help as he used to, and it's only five minutes before he's off and rolling to therapy. I take a lot longer. This morning it's taking even longer than usual, though, and she is surprisingly quiet and thoughtful during the whole process. I wait for her to say something. Instead, she seems distracted and distant. Finally, I can't stand it any longer, and I have to say something. Indeed, one of my glaring faults. I'm not big on silence unless I know you real well. "What?"

"What, what?" she asks.

"What are you thinking about? It's painfully obvious something is bugging you. You've been quiet since you came in here this morning." Classic transference at its finest. The patient has become the doctor. But everybody needs someone who will listen to them, whether it's the nurse dressing them, the therapist urging them to do one more rep on the weight machine, or the psychiatrist himself. (I think psychiatrists are the most notoriously screwed up of the bunch, but that's another story.) So, in the hospital, you end up getting close to the people whose job it is to see to your needs. It's not intentional or preplanned. All you have to do is show an interest, feigned or otherwise, and people will go out of their way to tell you about themselves. No problem is too large or too small. Bring it on. Pam was not going to be the exception.

"I hope you and your wife make it," she says, deflecting it back to me. Emotional ping pong, I love it.

"Yeah, me too, but what's that got to do with the price of rice? Now, what's really on your mind?"

"I think Peter and I are going in separate directions," she finally says, despondent, not looking for a reply, just letting something go that she had held onto for far too long. I notice only half of her earrings are in today, if that matters. They still number about eight. I'm into piercings and tattoos (even though I don't have one). They all seem to tell a story about an individual.

"You don't buy into the whole religion thing, is that it?" I counter.

"That and I just get the impression he's leaving me behind."

"Leaving *you* behind? Shouldn't it be the other way around? After all, you've got more to offer him than he has to offer you," I say, thinking this is good solid advice.

"You can be a total ass, you know that? If that's what you think, how can you imagine that you and your wife will stick it out?"

"Gee, I hadn't thought of that. At least not in the last ten minutes." It's all I had been thinking about since I woke up. My wife was young, attractive, selfish, and a sexual predator. Maybe that's the wrong word, but she definitely likes being in the spotlight and garnering the attention of men.

"If you don't mind me asking," I say, "which means I'm going to ask anyway, and you can answer if you like. Why the hell did you marry Peter in the first place? Okay, you're no spring chicken and granted, there are better-looking nurses out there, and you could stand to lose a couple of pounds here and there, and a trip to the gym once a week—"

"Okay, okay, enough already. Fuck you. What's your point?"

"Simply that *you* could do better. Why put yourself through the hassle of hangin' with a Quad if you don't have to?" I am pushing this topic as far as I can because the similarities between Pam and Peter and my wife and I are in the same ballpark, and I crave information. My wife and I will be right where Peter and Pam are at this moment, give or take the religious aspect, and the thought is unnerving.

"First, I don't think of it as 'hanging with a Quad.' As I said before, he's my husband, and I don't see his disability. I mean, it's there, but it's not what defines him. At least, that used to be the case. Now it seems he's backpedaling, looking for crutches or something. After all these years, I thought he was over the labels and the stereotypes, but he's suddenly back in mourning over the loss of his mobility, or he can't wait to overexplain his situation. He's craving uniqueness or something."

"Well, that makes sense to me. Rest assured, I realize I'm a rookie, but do you ever seriously think you get over the loss of your mobility?"

"I honestly don't know. I like to think you get over it, and then maybe something comes up. It's a miracle cure, a biological clock ticking loudly, or maybe it just gets bigger the longer you try to ignore it, but I'm rethinking that whole part about 'the chair doesn't define you.'"

"That isn't what I want to hear. I want to hear that it just gets easier, and there are pots of gold at the end of every fucking rainbow."

"You know," she says as she plunks herself down on the corner of the bed. That corner of the bed is getting a workout. It becomes apparent that physical therapy has been put on hold this morning. So now we're just sharing. Big yay for me so far because an honest discussion trumps therapy.

"Do go on," I encourage her.

"When Peter and I first got together, it was a hell of a lot easier," she continues, settling in, "and I had more patience to deal with a Quad and all their never-ending demands, but it just plain wears you down over the years. I mean, before, when we were first going out, no hill seemed too big to push up. Challenges were an accepted daily part of our lives. Now it seems like every molehill is a mountain, and all the daily rituals and hardships are wearing me out. Maybe it's because I deal with this shit in the hospital all day," and she spreads her arms, encompassing what I imagine is the whole seventh floor, "and then I go home and do it all over again. If you want free advice, whatever you and your wife do, accept all the help you can get. This wheelchair thing is too huge for one or two people to deal with all at once. You have to spread it around. It can't become bigger than the both of you."

"Why don't I just slit my wrists right now and get it over with?"

"Stow it, Wagner. You're not that type. All I'm saying is that it just becomes a huge obstacle after a while. All the preparations and worrying about shit like 'routine' days and bad days, accessible and inaccessible, bowels or bladder, flat tires, and limp dicks. I'm just getting sick of the whole mess."

"Wait, go back. Flat tires and limp dicks?" It figures that those two are the only things I heard. The rest was just blah, blah, blah.

"Okay, you didn't need to hear that last bit, but it's all part of the package. It all adds to the frustration. It just seems so futile."

"It sounds like someone isn't getting enough credit. What do you want? Some kind of above and beyond the call of duty medal for putting up with a Quad? You married the bugger. You could have walked away, literally and figuratively, but you decided to get married instead. I don't feel sorry for you. You made your bed, so now you have to lie in it or get a new fucking bed."

"It's not that easy."

"Bullshit, why is it not that easy?"

"I love him," she says with a small sigh. And now I'm a little gobsmacked by the shift in direction.

"Does he love you?" I don't think I have ever asked this question of anyone before. Certainly never sober, that's for sure. It's getting deep for me, and she is a real buzzkill.

"I think so, but between you and me, Quads might not be capable of loving anyone because they're so caught up in themselves. They define their whole world through their disability."

"And yet you say you don't define him through his disability. You're confusing the shit out of me. So, what, you've accepted it better than him?" I'm rethinking this whole ball of wax. Physical therapy ain't looking so bad right now. Yanking on weights beats pulling heartstrings and playing mediator.

"Yeah, that's exactly what I'm saying. I'm okay, and Peter's not okay. He wants more and more attention. It's like he's put himself above mere mortals. He associates being a Quad with being special. It's a fraternity, and you have to be a Quad to understand another Quad. Other people, *normal people*, need not apply. If I hear 'How could you begin to relate?' one more time, I might bring him to the hospital and get Wes to smother him with a goddamned pillow."

"Need I point out how well that turned out? But getting back to Quads feeling 'special,' I'm a Quad, and I don't feel this way, at least I don't think I do. In fact, I feel spectacularly unspecial."

"You're new at this. Wait until you get out there in the real world."

"Everybody always says that. It's like that while I've been in the hospital, the world has changed or something. It's the same fucked-up interesting world as far as I'm concerned. I'll just find it a little harder to get where I'm going. I'll never look at stairs or toilets the same way again, but I'll still be the same guy."

"You know what, I'm going to slowly step away from the bed and pretend we never had this conversation. Maybe you won't change, who knows. On the other hand, so far you don't act like a special case Quad, so perhaps there's hope for you. My advice would be to steer away from other wheelchair people."

"Hey, that's what I was thinking. It is pretty fucked up advice, though, because I am a wheelchair person."

"Oh no, you're not, at least not yet. Believe me when I say this." She seems pretty adamant.

"I guess I'll have to take your word for it."

"For now, but you've got plenty of time to find out everything firsthand. You already belong to the fraternity."

"And I'd give up my membership in this fraternity in a New York minute." It's as if she thinks this 'being in a wheelchair thing' was a conscious decision.

"You and your wife should be having this conversation," she says with finality, and I can tell this conversation has wound its way down, and I close my eyes to pretend I am almost asleep. It seems that going to sleep is my chosen escape plan.

"You're absolutely right," I agree, but I knew that my wife and I wouldn't be having this conversation any time soon. We weren't ready. It was painfully evident to me that *our* relationship would be drastically different, and it didn't make sense to point all this out to my wife, or Pam for that matter. At this juncture, I was depressed, and I did go back to sleep, hating my new life.

CHAPTER THIRTY-THREE

STEPS TWO AND THREE: BARGAINING AND THEN ANGER. I'M GOING BACKWARDS

DAY ONE HUNDRED AND TWO with no relief in sight. I'm marooned on a small island with no chance for rescue. It is a memorable day—a benchmark day! This was the arbitrary day, my actual deadline for "sparing"—getting feeling back in new and different places of my body. Alas, this was not the case, as I had suspected in the first month.

My body has read up on the spinal cord separation handbook, and it is following the script right down to the letter. So let me see: No triceps, check. No inside forearm muscle, check. Arm wrestling career put on hold, check. No feeling at all below the shoulders. Check fuckity check.

Conversations are still all questions with no answers. We are all assembled (the crew) in our smoking pit, sipping "real coffee" from the nurse's station that's laced with scotch. Mr. Mawani's tragic legacy (wherever he may be) is free booze. Wes went through all of Mawani's personal belongings before the family got there—because he's just Wes—and he found four sixty-pounders of scotch in his little wardrobe. Everyone has their own "private" desk and drawer combination and a wardrobe closet where they keep their regular and personal shit. I've got cashews, dental floss, a couple of bucks for expenses (nurse coffee fund), and clothing hanging in the wardrobe. You know, just regular stuff, casual clothes—and by that I mean one button-up shirt, two sweatshirts, two hoodies, and three pairs of various colored sweatpants. Clothes don't matter much to Quads. Functional is the rule of the day, but not so with Mr. Mawani. He had no clothes to speak of. Although he had a suit in there (getting dressed for his own funeral), he had no cashews or dental floss, and he didn't drink coffee, but the man did drink scotch, lots of scotch, a real game-changer for the fucked-up five—Wes, Young Dean, Scott, Carl, and myself. We've all had a buzz going on. Assorted prescription drugs and booze will do that for you. Demerol and scotch are my two favorite things this week, last week, and the week before. It doesn't get better than this up on the seventh floor.

"You can still have sex, right?" It starts. It always starts this way with Young Dean.

"Yeah, sure, why not? You're just missing your legs, not your dick," answers Wes, exasperated.

"And you can still use your hands?"

"Yeah, I guess so. Fuck it, Dean, just answer the question. You keep complicating this goddamn game," I chime in.

"You're sucking the fun out of it," says Wes. We are, of course, all playing the "What's Better Sweepstakes," only it's taken on new dimensions. Nothing is cut and dry anymore. We're all becoming cagey veterans when it comes to profit and loss. There aren't any absolutes unless they're specified.

"So, you could, you know?" says Young Dean, giving his hand a couple of shakes. He is still not satisfied with what his choices might be.

"Oh, for Christ's sake," I interject, "Yeah, you can wank, or jerk off, or whatever you want to do, all fucking day long if you want to." I have been the unofficial referee since the "Sweepstakes" started, which seems like a lifetime ago.

"Well, then I pick being a double leg amputee. No contest."

"What if a cure for spinal cord injuries came out in five years? You can't just ask for your legs back. You'd be sitting on your stumps, pulling your dick while the rest of us are walking around and pulling on our dicks," I point out while pouring another liberal shot of scotch.

"Big deal, five years is a long time to wait for a cure. You could get in a lot of wanking in that time." Young Dean is quite insistent on this point.

"Maybe to a seventeen-year-old who's still a cherry, but to a guy who started chicken-choking at eleven, five years isn't that big a deal," Wes says unnecessarily.

"All right, that's enough, Wes. Why do you find it necessary to torture Young Dean every time you play this game?" I ask, only because I was getting sick of listening to Wes and Young Dean, and I could feel Carl suffering silently beside me. Again, Carl rarely said much, although he did grumble a lot. Mostly he was a quiet, dour individual with a primarily bald round head and eyes that bored into you. Carl was like a white, pissed-off Charles Barkley, with a prominent brow and a wrinkled neck with skin folds rolled down his neck. He was a C6 Quad, which gave him a little more mobility than Young Dean, Scott, or myself, but he wasn't driven to improve. He silently and resolutely endured. However, this morning, while we were sitting around having coffee and booze in the smoking pit, Carl started to volunteer information.

He told us how he became a Quad in a logging accident, which was well known through the grapevine (large fucking grapevine in a hospital), and he was married with three kids. It took me two months to get that much information out of him. Nobody had ever met his kids, but I'd seen his wife a few times. She was rumored to be a matronly type, a good mother, a pleasingly plump woman who doted on him (Pam's words). She had taken over a lot of the hospital's care, even going as far as to assist in his routines. "Routines," once again, were what Quads, Paras, and nurses commonly called getting a suppository up your ass, getting stimulated by a digital finger, getting your colon cleansed, before putting on just another condom catheter and dressing for the day ahead. Carl had his routines in bed (finally figured that mystery out), refusing to suffer the indignity of sitting over the toilet on a commode chair or "crapping in public," as he called it. I applauded his wife for her efforts, but I couldn't see the reasoning.

I was a strong proponent of only asking my wife for help if all other options were exhausted. I figured that if you structured your life around

4 and ½ Steps

the care and feeding of a Quad, it would burn you out real fast. Peter and Pam, unfortunate names, were a constant reminder of that. The outside was still a lifetime away, and while there were nurses to take care of disagreeable functions, let them. Milk the system while you can. Yessiree, I think those very words should be a Quad battle cry. Anyway, this morning Carl had brought this up and not in a delicate way. That's what sparked the current game of the "What's Better Sweepstakes."

"My wife was trying to give me a blow job this morning," he said without preamble while we were all enjoying our morning fortified coffee, "and I felt nothing, absolutely nothing. She might as well have been sucking on my big toe. And about a week ago, she sat right on my face and almost smothered me. I couldn't even get a breath to yell for help. She ain't no lightweight, you know. I couldn't have lifted her off if I wanted to. And straight fucking is useless cause I'm always on the bottom, and I can't move or feel anything. I might have a hard-on, or maybe it went away. I couldn't tell. The goddamn things have a mind of their own. So, what could she be getting out of that? Besides, I hate the bottom. So basically, sex is a fucking write-off. What a miserable fucking life," and then Carl shut up again and refused to elaborate, not that elaboration was essential. Instead, it gave everybody sitting there enough fuel to keep their imaginations running full out for more than a couple of laps around the track, all except Young Dean. He was bursting with questions and fidgeting around until Wes engaged him in this current game of the "Sweepstakes" to put things into perspective. Double leg amputee or a useable regular dick. That was the question.

Carl just sat there mute after he gave us the update on his sexual proclivities, and he wasn't up for any games. A good thing, too, because the game's theme would change on a whim, and you had to keep up. In which position and where could you have sex? Where exactly was the amputation? Below or above the knee? This game might seem like a bleak and inappropriate waste of time, but we were all damaged fucking people trying to find our way in the dark. Young Dean and Wes were the leading players this morning. I was still trying to figure out how Carl managed to fit all this experimentation into his regular hospital regime. The biggest misnomer in the hospital was the term "privacy curtain," and he hadn't been off the seventh floor that I could recall. Maybe the nurses knew what was happening behind the curtain and chose to look the other way. My wife and I were content to wait until after being discharged. At least I was.

"The first roommate I had when they plunked me on the seventh floor," says Scott, joining in for the first time today and breaking me out of my semi-drunken reverie, "was a guy called Stan. Studly Stan, I called him. He was slightly brain injured, fell out of a pickup truck down some dirt road (Albertans are weird, every fucking injury story has a pickup truck in it), and landed on his head. Scrambled his brain a little, but he wasn't quite in Thomas's league. Anyway, he accidentally poured a kettle of hot water on his feet and had to come back to the hospital. Nice enough guy, harmless really, but all he did all day and all night was jerk off. No shit," and he sees me looking at him with my eyebrow raised skeptically, so he elaborated. "I mean, he'd sleep and eat and stuff, but leave him alone for five minutes, and he'd be doing the five-finger shuffle, the jizz handshake, you know what I mean?"

"Nice picture," I say, unwilling to get into this. My imagination had enough to deal with, but a drunk Scott wouldn't let it go, and Wes and Young Dean were a captive audience.

"How many times a day?" asks Young Dean, with something sounding almost akin to envy, not idle curiosity.

"I don't know for sure," says Scott. "I mean, I didn't count or anything, but fifteen, no, twenty times a day sounds about right."

"Fuck that," says Wes. "Nobody can beat off twenty times a day. Maybe in my prime, I could do ten."

Scott was undeterred. "Hey, this guy just had no stop in him. It's all he did. His dick must have been super-fucking human. Mine would be all scraped raw and red after about five."

"Fuck me, you guys are killing me," I finally say, "I'm going to go for a push around." I had a good buzz on, and I was getting a little better at pushing. I used the wheels to propel the chair forward, fuck the outside rails. Suitable for Rick Hanson but useless for a Quad, and I had pushed the chair around enough on floor seven to give me some confidence in my meager pushing ability. You betcha, a few laps of the floor, probably 100 yards all the way around, past the elevator where the old folks hung out, around a corner, forty more yards straight, around another corner, repeat until your shoulders burn. This small feat was all well and good, but I needed a more significant test.

I hit the button for floor number one; thank Christ I could now hit the control buttons, and down I went. I took a left at the elevators (turning right took you to therapy) and started pushing down a hallway. About fifty yards down, I hit the magic Quad button that opened doors automatically, and I was suddenly in an old unused part of the hospital. It smelled musty.

It was straight-up eerie. There was not a soul around. It was like a long echo chamber, and I could hear myself breathe. Nevertheless, I pushed along, noting in my mind that the entire world was not all level and paved with linoleum, unfortunately, so this was relatively easy. It was a brave new world out beyond the doors, but I felt like an explorer, for now, sitting back and enjoying the ride, easy peasy.

The doors worked just fine. Next, I went through another door that stayed full-on open for twenty seconds, and I went straight on another fifty yards. That's when I came to a small hurdle, my first real test. There were five stairs in front of me, and beside the stairs was a ramp. The ramp went to the left for about ten feet, the equivalent of two and a half stairs, right to a lovely little landing area, a level spot where you could turn your chair and go up the next ramp to the top. It was five stairs in all, a total height all told of three and a half feet. This little exploit should be a snap, I'm thinking, although it's the first ramp I've encountered when there wasn't someone else doing the pushing. No one around to see me succeed or fail, nobody but me.

I took about a four-foot run over even ground to get me up to speed, and took another push when I got about a third of the way. I then took another with considerable effort to get me within one foot of the landing area. It was right then that gravity laughed at me. I was trying for one last finishing push. One big try, "Over the top boys," but instead, I had just enough strength to hold me in that one spot. I tried, I really fucking tried, but I couldn't move another inch. I was stuck in limbo, no up or down. It was all I could do to hold myself in place. If I reached for the brakes, I would succumb to the inevitable pull of that laughing fuckface gravity. I hung on, neither going up nor down for what seemed like an hour but was probably ten minutes. I could feel my shoulders burn, and my arms started to shake. The level ground was right there.

I thought about a guy from the TV show *Survivor,* of all things. He climbed up a large pole with notches on it every two feet. Six people were holding onto their poles. The last guy hugging the pole without touching the ground won immunity, and they were safe and couldn't be voted off the Island. Four people out of the six were taken out early, one grudging foot at a time, yet two guys stuck to the top of this fifteen-foot pole like they were hugging heaven. Both had their eyes closed, never moved a muscle, and sweat was pouring out of them as the day's heat took its toll. They stayed that way for forty minutes, neither giving an inch, until one of them opened his eyes and adjusted his grip, sliding down two feet and again holding on for dear life. Another twenty minutes passed, and finally, the guy that adjusted started slipping slowly downward, but the one skinny guy never missed a beat. It was like he was made of stone. He was the last man up the pole and had only slid a foot down. He was the winner, and when he released his grip and slid down, he was totally exhausted. He couldn't even stand by himself, and his skin was red and abraded down his whole body like someone had taken sandpaper to him.

I was channeling that guy. I was not going to move one fucking inch.

That's when Isaac Newton played his trump card, and the law of gravity made my hand slip, almost imperceptibly and just enough so that I was slipping sideways a half-inch at a time. My only option was to release my other hand to stay straight. Inch by agonizing inch, I lost the challenge. I finally held up my hands and let the chair take me, and take me it did. I was almost back on level ground when the left wheel hit the side of the stair rail.

I flipped right backward and smoked my head on the linoleum that I used to love; excellent for pushing, shithouse lousy for landing on. I blacked out, briefly saw stars, felt the sharp numbing pain in my neck, and without further exploration, I knew the stitches that they put in my head three and a half months ago had opened up, the scar itself had parted, and when I did reach up, I had a generous amount of blood on my hand. So I just lay there as the pain subsided, or I just got used to it, and I rethought that whole idea of going solo.

They found me one and a half hours later, laying in blood with a broken baby finger bent right in half that, fortunately for me, I couldn't feel. A janitor found me. He pushed the panic button, and they whisked me back upstairs to my bed, stitched my broken eggshell head together, and of course, scheduled an X-ray for the next day. I generally laid there unresponsive and contrite, feeling vulnerable and broken. They finally loaded me up with drugs and closed the curtain around me. I mention this because before I could blissfully close my eyes as the drugs were doing their thing, I cried for the first time (maybe the second time). The tears wouldn't stop. I thought of my wife and what she must be going through. I thought of my parents, who undoubtedly had expectations from their eldest son. I cried because my family and friends would never look at me the same again. I cried out of self-pity, gut-wrenching, bitter, teeth-clenching self-pity. At some point, I must have gone to sleep. I vaguely remember someone changing my pillow and turning me sideways. There was no pain, just a feeling that I had fallen off a cliff, only falling, no happy ending where I hit bottom and died, or that this was all a bad dream. Even in the darkest recesses of my brain, it kicked in. I knew then that I would never walk again.

CHAPTER THIRTY-FOUR

STEP TWO: JUST FLAT-OUT ANGER

DAY ONE-TWENTY, OR CLOSE TO that. Rinse, repeat. It's fucking *Groundhog Day*, except Bill Murray could transform his life and learn something new every day in that movie. In this movie, I am permanently stuck in neutral. I wake up and eat four boiled eggs—they can't mess that up. They're hard-boiled every time with egg yolks you could bounce, but I knew what I was getting. Then they dress your ass. I stare at Arlene, talk to Pam, and ogle Monique: I had another nurse crush. Vince the upright Para is still going with her, and he drops by now and then to smoke a joint and give us tales of the outside world. He seems genuinely concerned about my bad attitude, and I can see why. I've been in an electric wheelchair since I failed the stair climb. Now I'm seat-belted like a child in a car seat, wheelie bars attached that goes a steady four miles an hour. I slow down when taking a corner, stop slowly, turn switchbacks even slower, and follow the hallway rules. There are fucking limitations.

The electric wheelchair gives me the power to get out of my room and away from the hospital. It lets me go out to the only restaurant close to the hospital with my brother, sisters, mother, father, and wife. Excellent change of scenery and food, but my brother looks distraught at all times. I was the one supposed to protect his ass, watch his back, and wade right in swinging for the fences. He lives in Fort St. John, and there is no end to the riggers, rednecks, cowboys, and Indigenous Peoples that don't consider it a fill-your-boots-night until someone goes home with a missing tooth and a black eye or two. You've got to look around before you start swinging, but just add rye whiskey, and my brother can be an instant asshole, and I'm not far behind (I learned early to pace myself during fight nights). You can't win 'em all, but we had a pretty good record of wins and losses.

Anyway, you're up to date in the world of sports. I've got to change the channel on that part of my life, only it's hard to do, and I can't seem to shake it off. Move on, buddy, you're not going to be swinging for the fences again, but the unfortunate position of being in a chair is that it can't change you completely in every aspect. I can still be a drunk asshole, which is unfair to anyone because who would hit a Quad?

Too many random thoughts, especially with family or friends around, and nothing feels comfortable and easy anymore. I feel like I have to entertain them. My thoughts jump around like a coked-up frog on an electric lily pad. There is no end to wheelchair salesmen (and saleswomen) that want you to buy their shit. I'm having a hard time picking a chair type for the rest of my life. Quickie, Pride, Invacare . . . and they're like used car salesmen. This chair does this, and this one can go "five" miles an hour. This one comes with a drink holder (a practical option for me), and currently, I was testing a Quickie when it happened. The "I can still be an asshole" part.

We were all sitting in the smoke room one night because unless someone bitches heavily, Quads will not go downstairs to smoke, even though the rules have been changed since we've been there. So it was Scott, Carl, Young Dean, Wes, and Vince the upright Para, who had come for a visit. We drank the last of Mr. Mawani's scotch, straight up and warm. I was reading a comic book with my back to them, *Daredevil, Spiderman,* not sure which, and someone (I put that one on Vince the upright Para) flicked a switch on the back of the chair, and you'd think the whole place was on fire. Sirens, lights, and my joystick lit up like a Christmas tree. They were laughing their collective asses off, and I just casually rolled out, headed for the nurse's station, and had someone turn it off. I think it was Althuna, but back I went, pretty as you please, as if nothing happened. I casually rolled back into the smoke room without a word and pulled back under the table to continue reading my comic book.

What does my good friend Doug Walker (Wok) always say? He was a steady influence in my old Maple Ridge life, and he always said, "Fool me once, shame on you, fool me twice, shame on me," and that very thought crossed my mind when they flipped the switch the second time (I put this one on Scott), and it was another fire drill and another joke on me. My eyes went black, and they watered with frustration. I've been told that happens when I lose my shit, and I had lost my shit. I calmly turned the wheelchair onto full speed, four fucking miles an hour (the salesman assured me), and I reversed the chair right into the whole fucking pack of them. They were gathered in the corner by the window, three pushchairs, one electric chair, and Vince the upright Para sitting on the table with his walking sticks. I rammed into them with the beautiful soul-satisfying crunching sound of breaking chairs and metal twisting, with people yelling "What the fuck?" Knowing that I could just "power" away without a scratch-made me smile. It felt so good that I came forward another four feet and did it again. My joystick was lit up like the fourth of July, and the chair was emitting a *weeoo, weeoo* noise that was loud enough to be heard at the nurse's station. I might have even done it again, but the Quickie finally got tangled in the jumble of people and busted wheelchairs, and my Quickie wasn't so quickie anymore.

The sirens and the lights were still in full-on panic mode, but I never said another word. Wes started yelling his head off, cursing my skinny Quad ass to hell and back until two nurses and a janitor came running (what is it with fucking janitors? There must be a million of them working at this place, and they follow me around to clean up my messes). In the end, it was a very satisfactory result. I bent one of Vince the upright Para's sticks in two, broke Young Dean's wrist (yeah, jerk off with that motherfucker), and Scott's wheelchair footrests were scrap metal. His shin would be X-rayed later for breakage, and it turned out to be a greenstick fracture to the tibia—a shin bone—I'm told, and he was sporting a clumsy-looking cast the next day. Carl came out relatively unscathed, and he had a giant smile on his face, a satisfied Cheshire Cat fucking grin (Carl freaks me out), and it took them a good ten minutes to untangle everybody and pick up the pieces. Wes swore at me for the whole ten minutes and mentioned various scenarios of where and how he would "fucking kill me," something everyone yells when the fight is already lost. My expression never changed. I didn't say a goddamned word, and they pushed my broken, still-scream-ing-like-an-ambulance-stuck-in-traffic Quickie wheelchair back to my room and chucked me in bed. Someone found the switch and turned it off eventually. Blessed silence reigned.

I lay in bed with my eyes leaking, replaying the last half hour in my mind, and decided I would do it again if the opportunity arose even though these were "my people," my "partners in crime," the only ones who might genuinely understand me by virtue of their damaged spinal cords. I had come to know them all in my stay at the hospital. I had seen them at their best and their worst. It was Vince the upright Para who finally broke into my reverie as he parted the privacy curtains with his forearm crutch—the one left undamaged. I was sure I would get the Mr. Mawani treatment; only beaten half to death with an aluminum crutch instead of a sturdy cane, but Vince the upright Para was smiling and chuckling at the same time.

"Holy shit, man, that was a fine game of bumper cars or chicken or whatever you want to call it," he finally said. "You can bet your ass there's a broken bone or two in that bunch."

"You aren't going to beat the fuck out of me with your crutch?" I said, looking around for a place to hide. A place that didn't exist. But Vince the upright Para surprised me with his following comment.

"No chance. Why would I do that?" he said, taken aback. "I would have done the same damn thing. Young Dean and Scott flipped your switch, literally and figuratively." Maybe there was more to Vince the upright Para than I had initially thought. I had him pegged as a redneck, a dopey dude, the kind of guy you would find at every demolition derby or monster truck rally with a hard hat that had two beers attached to its sides, one straw sticking out of his mouth. He sat down on the edge of my bed, gave me a semi-serious look, and started talking.

It was like being on Santa's lap. He patted my legs first, knowing full well I wouldn't feel it, and he sighed audibly. "Look, Wag, I've seen the real world, the outside, the world you inherit when you get out of this freakin' asylum, and it ain't pretty. I have sticks, man. I can take the stairs and hit the head if I have to, but you, my friend, can't. You will get stared at and questioned incessantly about how you got to be in a wheelchair, and anybody with a brother, sister, or uncle in one will *understand* how you feel. There will also be the 'comparison guys.' You know those who tell you their sad-ass stories about how they were briefly paralyzed and recovered or still had problems. People will put their hands gently on your shoulder and tut-tut like they know how you feel or what you're going through, and I know how much you hate being touched—you're a little weird about that, but that's your prerogative. I'm just saying that you will have to dial it down a notch."

"I'm trying to, man," and I don't know where the tears came from, but they ran freelance down my cheeks. I sniffed my nose, shook my head slightly, and pulled it together. "I'm just flat out fucking scared, Vince, and that doesn't sit well. I hate people in wheelchairs, and I know that's just screwed up, as they are my friends through circumstances. I know I should be on board with this shit, but I want to scream every goddamn morning when I get up and come out of a good Demerol dream, and it occurs to me that I'm a fucking cripple. This frustrates every fiber of my being." I felt wrung dry after that revelation.

"You realize, though, that you're the one to blame. You put yourself there. You made stupid choices, and this is the result." He then squeezed my dead, unfeeling foot, got up, and gave a little laugh while he shook his head. "I can't wait to see you in a couple years. Your attitude is going to eat you up inside."

"You know what?" I said, sighing myself and compartmentalizing my emotions.

"'Kay, I'll bite. What?"

"I wish you would have just beat the fuck out of me with your crutch." Then there was an uncomfortable silence until I softly suggested he go suck a dog dick. I added, unnecessarily, "If I see you coming, I'll turn my chair around and wheel away as fast as I can," which was funny because my "fast as I can" is still about as fast as a baby can crawl. Vince the upright Para had beat Young Dean in the big hallway challenge. He outraced (out crutched) Young Dean, who had his power chair, in a twenty-foot show-down. It was quite a thing to witness. I might have said something else, but we were rudely interrupted. Wes had finally made his way back to his bed with one wheel that was so bent up it barely turned.

"Wagner, you fuck. You useless piece of shit. I'm gonna cave your fucking skull in. I'm going to find a truck and run you the fuck over, twice, backward and forwards," and he was spitting as he said it with wild-eyed abandon. I made a serious mental note that I would stay as far away from Wes and his imaginary truck as possible for a while. But I knew Wes prob-ably better than anyone else in this god-cursed hospital, and I knew he'd get over it, and we would have a good laugh about it after another semi-drugged-out sleep. After all, I hadn't broken *his* bones, and his wheelchair was a rental, so no harm, no foul. Vince the upright Para, still chuckling, turned and left, twisting his whole body sideways, laying his full weight on the one crutch, and somehow spinning his body forward. That son-of-a bitch would walk upright no matter how many obstacles you put in his way.

The following day, Wes wasn't in his bed, presumably away at therapy or off to the eighth floor for a different type of therapy. They had removed my busted-up, squeaky, super annoying power chair sometime during the night, and I never saw the Quickie salesman again, probably a good thing in hindsight because Invacare had a better product; a tank of a chair that suited me just fine.

I woke up slowly, replaying last night's shenanigans over in my head until Pam came in and dressed me without a word, save a terse "Good morning." She then informed me that I was summoned to another meeting. As usual, all the nurses had come together on a shift change to discuss the progress of the general population, and I was number one on the Hit Parade that morning.

Once again, I was brought in front of the school principal without counsel or backup. It was just me, *Doctor Doom*, and three angry-looking nurses; Pam, Monique, and the Charge Nurse (who had been instrumental in untangling everyone after the smash-up); and surprisingly, the Physio along with the Occ-Doc (the occupational therapist). They were obviously upset with me. Apparently, they expected *more* of me, like I was some kind of pet project or star pupil that had gone astray, an experiment gone awry. I find this funny because almost every teacher I've had from Grade Four to my last year of university had the same disappointed look on their collective silly faces. A look that said, "You can do better than this," or "You're not living up to your potential, so wipe that smug smile off your face." Okay, that last one was more of a high school thing. In college or university, they ask you to rewrite shit or overthink shit, and if you refuse, they stick you with a C-plus, which was always a fine mark by my way of thinking. It put me right smack dab in the middle of the rat race without expending pointless energy to be something I wasn't.

"So, I'm a C-plus, right?" I had to ask, but Pam, the Physio, and Occ-Doc looked skeptical. "So, a solid C?" I ventured. Thumbs down from Pam, and I quit guessing. "Aw, c'mon, man. I just don't feel like rolling around on a mat some mornings, and sure, occupational therapy is practical and all, but practicing how to print your name, put on your clothes, and pick shit up from a dime to a coffee cup is somewhat demeaning."

"We will cut back on your Demerol dose," said Hilda, the Charge Nurse who had made no impression on me save for that last statement.

"Hold your horses. You mean, like completely?" I ask, incredulous, as this is my favorite thing about hospital living. This is the juice, the oil that stops the gears from grinding. I was addicted to the stuff. I knew it, and they knew it. So, yep, they went straight to the jugular.

"Mr. Wagner, we have accommodated you for too long. From now on, you will receive a small dose of Demerol meant to wean you off gradually, and then a small dose of Ativan when necessary. You are treating this hospital as your personal playground, and that stops today," and it was almost as if she was gloating, like she had accomplished something. I couldn't help but think she had been waiting for the walls to cave in around me, wanting me crushed by them.

"Fine, fuck you." How far I had fallen; this was my best comeback. It was a gang beating, and in retrospect, it was a long time coming. But it was the big-time wake-up call. I guess I was forced to try harder to get the hell out of the hospital from here on in. No more busted knees and busted people.

"We'll see about that, Mr. Wagner."

"Yes, we will. I don't much like threats, and I don't do addiction," and that was that. It ended the *meeting*. Everyone gathered their papers together, *Doctor Doom* included, and walked by me and out the door. It seemed like the *Real World*, as Vince the upright Para had so aptly named it (because that's the way I thought about it too), had rudely arrived, and I was going to have to be a part of it whether I liked it or not. I wasn't that worried about the drugs or the nurses I had come to depend on. I didn't have an addictive streak in me. I could quit things and people in a minute, good or bad, but I was afraid of the real world and the rest of my bloody life, of fitting in, of being a part of it, diminished and small.

CHAPTER THIRTY-FIVE

RECOVERY, NOT A STEP, JUST TIME WELL SPENT

SO HERE I AM ON day one-twenty-nine or something, lying in bed still stoned. It's early, and the drugs haven't worn off yet. At least I still get some Demerol to sleep and a small dose (by my standards) of Ativan. It was a little harder kicking Demerol than I thought. There was lots of sweating, tossing and turning, and feeling sick. But it was worse than quitting cocaine (another story for another time). I watch the giant grade school clock tick off seconds. I'd kind of forgotten about the damn thing, and somehow, it was ticking way too loud. It's six a.m., and I can hear Wes snoring like a fucking bear because they doubled his drugs so he would stop coming up with new ways to end my life. I don't know how someone that small makes that kind of noise, and it isn't a consistent noise, not like Bob's boiling kettle. It's a hitching sound like he's drowning, and then it stops, but when you think he might finally be dead, he starts up again like an old man gargling gravel. Actually, Wes's spine was screwed up beyond my imaginings. Ramming Wes did not contribute to his failings. He just flat out had way more screws than me and a stainless-steel rod keeping more than a couple of vertebrae straight. Somehow, his steel rod had come unscrewed and he was suffering through a setback. He didn't talk about it much. Wes was not an over-sharer about his condition.

It is a beautiful day. The sun is coming through the windows, revealing all the dingy yellowness of the room, the cobwebs in the corners, and the flies (I've lately developed a "thing" about flies), some dead and some lazily struggling away, all caught up in them—so many comparative situations. I wonder what step those flies are experiencing? The one struggling, he just got snared, and I'm betting he's going through denial. I'm getting the hang of this shit. Anyway, I can feel the warmth on my face. Enjoy the sun, Wagner, and thank goodness for small miracles. Save that feeling for another "Sweepstakes" day. What's better? Beating off or feeling the sun on your face? That one ought to blow Young Dean's mind.

The sun feels so good, and I can close my eyes for a moment and go on a holiday in my mind. I glance at the big clock again, I can't help myself, and it's still early. The clock reads seven-thirty-four. The dust motes swim silently in the warm air, orchestrated by a puff of wind, and the hospital is quiet. It's a beautiful moment, but I can smell the piss and the Dettol as I'm lying here. It's an insistent smell, and I realize that I'm part of it, part of the cogs, gears, and smells that add to the daily grind of hospital life.

I know it's me that smells like piss. It isn't the first time, and it won't be the last. Although I barely notice it, fucking condom catheters, the mileage of these things is like trying to get five hundred thousand no-nonsense miles out of a Pinto. It just ain't going to happen. So, they will take another condom (I don't know what else to call it), and they will roll it down my dick, which is just trying to escape the whole undignified process, and then they will wrap the tape around the bottom, pulling up your flaccid "dick-skin." It's supposed to hold on, warrantied for one whole day, but it falls off or rips off when you move (hair removal at its worse), and then you piss yourself—way to spoil the start of a good day. There has to be something better, but this is why we are at a crossroads. The doctor wants your bladder to work naturally, voiding all the piss out of your body. The catcher bag is there, and I can see it one-quarter full and happy to receive a little more. "Bring it on," it's saying, and I've got another half-gallon of room to spare.

So, your bladder works naturally—yay for my bladder. You're just soaking the bed every time you void (a hospital term used way too often). Also, for some reason, you sweat your ass off like you're sitting in a fucking sauna drinking tea while you're sweating off last night's whiskey. This process is demeaning and degrading, but it's all part of the beautiful recovery process. Recovery, my ass. Fuck you, recovery. Moods are sure fickle in a hospital. Maybe I should get out of this place.

CHAPTER THIRTY-SIX

STEP FOUR: MORE DEPRESSION, IT PERVADES

SHUFFLE WAY AHEAD TO DAY one-hundred-and-fifty. Five inglorious months. My wife now works a full schedule of shifts at the Keg. She comes in sporadically, as she works nights, and when and if I see her, it is usually around three or four in the afternoon.

"Oops, got to get to work. Where did the time go?" my wife says.

And I say, "Okay, sweetheart, have a great shift, see you later." It sucks because you are helpless with making money, and she's out there waiting tables while I'm in here twiddling my thumbs (so to speak). It also sucks because I'm almost fresh out of visitors. After the first wave, the people cheering you on are getting on with their own lives. It's funny that it's what I wanted and why I insisted Calgary would be where I recovered, far away from the pitying eyes of friends and family. However, they haven't stopped cheering for me and wishing me the best. I do miss them, and I know they are there.

Since I've been here, the most remarkable thing was my friends getting together to have a "Wagner Donation Dance." They rented a hall, auctioned items off, charged for drinks, and took donations. It was somewhat degrading, but I had no choice. We were fresh out of vehicles, and taxis were far too expensive. So consequently, my friends—eleven hours and some six hundred miles away—had a dance. More than three thousand dollars was mailed out, from cheques to quarters, and the big cash envelope had "Wish you well" cards from people I knew, respected, and loved in my skewed way. Maybe I wasn't as big of an asshole as I thought. The author of that chapter was due to my affiliation with the Pitt Meadows Garage Slo-pitch team. I have five or six years of beautiful memories from hanging out with the coolest people I ever knew. Coached by two "Hippies," nicknamed Deuce and Rhea, with a shitload of brothers—the Weistras and the Nordquists, three of each, six total—and two tough little fuckers named Barry and Louie, and replacement parts. I know that sounds like a significant cluster-fuck, but somehow it all came together, and I will never forget what they did to help me out. Okay, maybe I shed more than a few tears.

The envelope bought us the Ford LTD, a boat of a car that was perfect for transporting Quads around. Unfortunately, I still wasn't good at transferring. Getting me into that behemoth via transfer board and hard lifting was no small feat. Sometimes we would say, "Fuck the transfer board," and it became a complete weight shift transfer from a helper who could presumably move one-hundred-and-fifty pounds of bone and flaccid muscle. They would put my arms around their neck, lift and pivot, and sit me down again from chair to car. Adams excelled at it, as did Cousin Ken.

Cousin Ken showed up unannounced and almost unrecognizable one day, as I hadn't seen him since high school. He was a relative, not through marriage (I think I was related to half of Maple Ridge "through marriage"), but a blood relative. Ken's father was my grandmother's brother, my mother's uncle, and one of my father's best friends. My Uncle "Jock" was a Scotsman who had a family of three boys that lived five blocks away from us in Maple Ridge, and yet we only saw them at family reunions. The boys were close to my age. Ken was the youngest. Unbeknownst to me, he had moved from Maple Ridge to Calgary three years ago, was married, and had bought a house. Of course, I knew none of these things, which shows how much we kept in touch, but he was a bonus from day one.

He saw me two to three times a week on the seventh floor, and we watched the Toronto Blue Jays together. He loaded me into that old Ford

LTD what felt like a hundred times, going to his place for dinner or busting out of "gen pop" for late-night forays to bars and restaurants. Ken and his wife Liz figured hugely into my life.

On this particular morning, the paper-pusher Charge Nurse is not impressed. I wake up with a raging headache, a just-licked-a-rug feeling. I do this almost every second morning, and I take my broken body and swollen head down to therapy and give it my best shot. I've puked on the plastic mat more than once. Some people recover differently than others, puking is my "go-to" option some mornings, but you can sense she is getting really sick of my antics. I intuited this when she said, "Wagner, I am getting real sick of your antics. You are in a hospital, not a daycare. You either contribute to your recovery, or you can see the door, and I mean it." The last part was unnecessary because her face said, "I mean it," so it was a redundancy I endured.

Usually a smart-ass comment, a smirk, or a gesture would be my immediate response, but lately it feels like this situation is more of a hostage-taking. I say this because I believe I have Stockholm Syndrome; I have fallen in love with my captors. I can stay out late, piss myself, schedule my bowel care, get washed up, and get my daily prescription drugs. Then, finally, I get put in bed, and my laundry is taken care of by beautiful nurses who seem oblivious of my shenanigans—all except Pam.

"They will fire your ass out of here," she tells me one blurry morning, and she brings it on home with a harsh wake-up call. "You may think you're ready, but you're not even close. Is your apartment wheelchair accessible? Have you done any bathroom renovations? How are you going to take a shower? Who will take care of you when you get turfed out of here? Your wife has to work, and nothing comes for free. You've got to set up a home support system, pay them and train them, get in and out of your own fucking bed every night, have meals prepared, and get your own goddamn groceries. Someone has to change your catheter, clean you up, set you on a commode chair, brush your teeth, comb your hair, and get you into your electric fucking chair. You're going to wear out your welcome pretty quick around here if you haven't already, and you haven't done anything to prepare for your future. Not. One. Fucking. Thing." She finishes with a yell, followed by an audible sigh.

Well, let me tell you, that was a big-ass skull cruncher. It does, however, occur to me that Pam is right on all counts. I have only accomplished moving to a ground-floor apartment and buying a bath chair. Oh yeah, and I did decide on an electric wheelchair, but not the Quickie—the one with the alarm system—definitely not that one. Instead, it is an Invacare chair. I call it Bert. It goes four and a half miles an hour flat out. I have a shift knob on the left-hand side and a joystick for forwards and reverse on the right. It won't win any awards for esthetics, but it's a workhorse that weighs about three hundred pounds, and it feels substantial. It says this is a throne, and you are my vassals. At least, I tell myself this, but I don't feel like the king of anything. It sits in silent vigil at the side of my bed, waiting for me to get through my drug-induced, sometimes alcohol-fueled sleep every night, and then off we go again for a new adventure.

Pam has definitely made me think about my new life. She has flipped the pages. The Boston Pizza restaurant is opening in eight weeks, and I'm getting drunk and treating the hospital like a personal spa. All my needs are met; I'm bathed, get stuck on a commode chair when necessary, and get three squares a day. I have eaten one thousand chicken wings and fifty-two Salisbury steaks with a mysterious brown mushroom gravy. I have fallen into a rhythm, the repetitive boredom and structure that surrounds me has trapped me and has become my *new* life.

It is high time I finally put on my big-boy pants. I decided to set up my home for wheelchair access, cut back on the booze (cut back being a relative term), and meet with my Boston Pizza partners and the head office franchise people who helped me set up a restaurant from soup to nuts. I take advantage of my better-than-good friend Adams and his position at Boston Pizza as a setup guy to get the right mindset you need to prepare yourself for the grand opening. I had more or less worked at Boston Pizzas for years, doing the setup stuff and making enough pizza dough to feed an entire third-world country. Still, it is significantly different in your very own restaurant. You are ultimately held accountable at the end of the day for making your staff, your customers, and especially your partners feel satisfied, happy, and relaxed.

It is November, and I have stalled and got stuck in the mud. I have become institutionalized, and I guess a welcome to the real-world moment would eventually come, even though I was doing all I could to avoid it.

Wes, the long-haired wannabe rockstar, had left a couple of weeks ago. It was a sad day. We had a love-hate relationship, but he was my roommate through all the good times and hard times. He said, "It's been a big slice, choirboy," as he was going out the door. "I will leave you my tennis racquet. There are still plenty of flies and bees to smack." Somehow, that was the perfect thing to say, and I intuited that I might never see the little bugger again, which saddened me. Scott, the stoner, was gone without a goodbye (he never got over the "Quickie incident"), and Vince the upright Para came in less and less to smoke a joint and kick back on the eighth floor. Even Carl got his release papers, and he did come to my room to mutter a goodbye and even shake my hand for a long moment, wordless and stoic for three minutes, staring at me eerily and slightly smiling. It was like watching a pit bull smile while he's eyeing you up for a snack, and it was almost like he was trying to tell me something but he could not find the words.

He never found the words. At least he didn't find the *right* ones. Two weeks after he checked out, Carl ran his electric chair off a pathway, down an embankment, into the Bow River, all without a seatbelt, and he got swept downriver for a mile or two. I never went to his funeral, but I felt his pain. I was with him swimming (floating) downriver to his next adventure. I went on a monumental four-day binge when I heard about Carl. It was fucked up, and it fucked me up, bone-deep shit, stuff you just stored in your brain and thought about when the drugs wore off and the world got way too big. Why did you not ask for help, Carl? You fucking "Easter Island" statue.

And even Young Dean was making progress. His family had tricked out their basement into a wheelchair paradise. I'm sure they had staff in place to take care of his needs and as much home support as he needed, which was more than most. But unfortunately, Young Dean was still playing the "What's Better Sweepstakes" in his mind, and when we did meet up in the smoke room—neither one of us smoked—before he left, he had another new scenario.

"What would you pick?" he asked, still trying to justify or elevate his current circumstances, "being deaf, blind in one eye, and given only three weeks to live (he took Carl's death pretty hard too), or being right where you are now, in a damn wheelchair for life?"

"Fuck me, Dean," I finally said, "it was a time-waster, buddy. I dreamed it up in my twisted little mind, an exercise in perspective, not a goddamned blueprint for the rest of your miserable fucking life. You've got to let it go, man. It is what it fucking is, dude. Deal with it." And after that, I would pass him in the hallway, or see him in therapy rolling around on a mat or batting balloons around—we batted a lot of stinking balloons around. He would nod, and I would return his nod, and it again occurred to me right there that I did not like people in wheelchairs, not one little bit.

CHAPTER THIRTY-SEVEN

STEPS TWO AND FOUR: ANGER AND MAYBE DEPRESSION

I WAS STILL LOSING TRACK of days. Time rolled on, and really, the only day that seemed essential was my release date, which had finally arrived. It's past due. I'm deemed suitable for the outside world.

It was time to go, and I hadn't even tried to talk to the new guys. It's like a never-ending stream; they will never run out of new Quads and Paras to process. One interesting guy now lays in Mr. Mawani's old bed. His skin is almost ebony black, and he looks chiseled out of oak. He's in incredible shape. He looks like he could shit muscles, but he had a massive stroke. Go figure. At thirty-three years old, his previous life is now a memory. He has trouble talking, but he is the friendliest "mofo" you ever want to meet with a smile a mile wide.

A replacement for Vince. I feel sorry for him because most of the guys on the seventh floor, me included, fucked *ourselves* up while this guy just pulled a shitty card. Fate, kismet, karma, call it what you want. It just happens. Life is simply not fair sometimes. I wish I had just a touch of his positive attitude. He's the only guy I say goodbye to on my way out the door. Yes, it is graduation day. It's December twelfth. Six months, give or take, and I am finally out the door. My cousin Ken and my wife have come to collect me. I say goodbye to all the nurses who tried to make my life more liveable, and I appreciate them; I really do, but they have failed in their ministrations. I hate my fucking new life. I keep trying to find the positives, but I'm sucking at it. I want to rewind my life for six months. I want a mulligan, and I'll volunteer at a hospital, kiss babies, help old people, renounce my sins, apologize to all the people I've wronged, and then I stop and think. Whoa, there, Wag, it sounds like I'm going to go to an AA meeting, which is not the same. Never blame the booze. Being a Quad is not a lifestyle choice. It's hard getting kicked out of the nest. It's now Wagner versus the world. Maybe they helped me too much.

I took my time about it, getting my parole papers. I just know I'm not coming back. I ain't like Scott, Wes, Young Dean, Carl, or Vince the upright Para, who seem to draw some nostalgic moments out of returning and talking to the nurses and the new guys. That just isn't me. I won't need anyone else.

Total update, I am now paralyzed from just above the nipples down. I was so typical of a C5-6 Quad that they had even used me for teaching purposes. I laid naked in front of five interns at a time, who were poking at me with what looked like sharp chopsticks. They asked questions like, "Can you feel that? How about that? Where did you injure your spine?" I consoled myself, thinking the more people in research, the closer they would come to discovering a cure for spinal cord injuries. Remember, I was told by *Doctor Doom*, "It's an exciting time to be a Quad," and faint hope is better than no hope at all. Unfortunately, I often assumed that the "Cure was on the way."

So, my shoulders work. I could lift them up and down in a shrug. My arms were still useless, and the only feelings regained were in my thumb and index finger. Palms up, my wrist and arms were dead, but palms down (the knuckle side), I could lift my wrists. I could also see the outside of my forearm muscles flexing. Meanwhile, you could cut my leg off while I slept, and I wouldn't know it. I learned this the hard way later on—so many things to learn.

The first big lesson I learned on the outside is to stay out of hot tubs.

4 and ½ Steps

On the second day of my release, Rax (Ron Bignell) and his wife Debra, the head honcho for public relations or human resources at all CN Hotels across Canada, booked my wife and me into the Fairmont Hotel in Lake Louise. It was a bloody beautiful place, and we had luxury-laden adjoining rooms. Relax, drink champagne, and eat at a five-star restaurant, all on Debra's boss's dime. There just happened to be a hot tub in one of our rooms, so we drank more champagne than necessary and decided to go for the hot tub a couple of hours before dinner. First order of business, lift the Quad and lower him into the tub like dropping a big old egg in boiling water.

I distinctly remember my ass just went below the water line, and I was yapping about something inane (my specialty), and they dropped me in the rest of the way. All I recall was this massive headrush. As I was told later, I stopped mid-sentence and passed out cold, head on my chest, pure coma pass out.

Apparently, they lifted me out as quickly as I went in, and someone had the foresight to lay me in the bed and pack my body with ice packs, one on my head, a couple under my arms, and a few more around the rest of my body. I was out for about ten to twelve hectic minutes, and then I woke right up, felt great, and wondered what the hell had happened. Although my whole body was a bright red boiled lobster-like color, I felt relatively okay. Only my vision was a little off. Stars were floating everywhere. So I made a large note: don't do hot tubs. Bathwater can only be one hundred ten degrees, lower your body slowly into it, and don't drink a bottle of good champagne before bath time. We spent the next three days eating, drinking, cruising around Lake Louise, playing euchre late into the night, and everyone took care of me. I could have stayed there for a good month or more, but real life always gets in the way. Damn you, real life.

I have been out for five days now, and I am pleased to note that the apartment is not my enemy. I have a commode chair, a bath seat, a king-size bed, a pushchair, and Bert, the electric chair. I also have one random lady who answered my ad to take care of me. She was the only one who responded, but I didn't tell her that. She wouldn't have been my first choice. I can tell she's friggin' evil. She smells like old mothballs and wet wool. She rarely smiles, but my wife and I have to open the damn Boston Pizza. Any port in the storm.

I've got no beef with Boston Pizza. They are good at what they do. I've been in their shoes, helping people open Boston Pizza restaurants, and it's not fucking easy, especially if it's with a person who rarely goes to restaurants and never eats pizza, for that matter, and probably never will. I've been through this shit before when I was a walking guy. Grand openings rocked, and I couldn't wait for ours. Fortunately, I had already been to "Pizza School" with Kevin Lowe's sister (a hockey player, look it up), the Valalee's, Mike in particular, who knew more about pizza and how to run a restaurant than anyone alive or dead. He was *the guy*. He opened the franchise in Lethbridge, where I was headed that fateful night—what feels like a hundred years ago—and he did give the wife and me a job right on the spot while we waited for our restaurant to open.

Some stuff never changes, and opening a Boston Pizza is one of those things. It is a formula tried and true. It goes something like this. First, you pay a lot of money for the franchise name. Then you make big-time decisions about how many tables you want, including chairs for the restaurant and stools for the bar, the color scheme, the size of the T.V. in the lounge (I pushed for the largest giant screen I could find), and what kind of beer or wine you serve. The layout and kitchen are preplanned, so all Boston Pizzas are relatively the same. Most parts of the process are scripted and relatively easy.

Myself, I love the liquor reps. Who wouldn't? Labatt's, Bud, Canadian, Kokanee, and a dozen others are all vying for your nod to have access to the six or eight taps that serve draft. I went for eight beer taps and two wine taps, which was pretty much my most significant contribution, and let me tell you, it was a hard job picking which kinds of beer and wine I wanted to serve—lots of sampling and lots of freebies. I remember very little of it, except that at the end of all the "pickin's and choosin's" I had a large walk-in cooler full of free products, a new appreciation for craft beer, and a new respect for my wife. She put me to bed and put up with my hangovers for six days running while I tasted and sampled enough beer and wine to fill a bathtub or two. Of course, that's one of the last things you do before opening. First, you had to do the less exciting steps.

The only thing that made any of this possible, six days of drinking and feeling like shit, was that I finally scrapped the condom catheter. This is not a regular part of the restaurant opening, but it was life changing. Some Bozo should have been all over the options in the hospital, but it wasn't like that. Instead, it was, "Mr. Wagner, you must utilize the fucking torturous condom catheter because it helps your bladder void on its own," like that matters anymore. After all, I will never stand up and take a piss.

It might seem silly and straightforward unless you're a Quad. I finally learned from an old guy in a wheelchair I met in a Chinese restaurant (Quads are notorious for filling your head with useless information when you meet them) who told me that "indwelling" catheters would save a lot of hassle. That fellow Quad informed me that they could insert a catheter into the end of your dick, hence indwelling. It's an apparatus you change only once a month, one that continually drains and empties into a large plastic receptacle that sits in a bag attached to the back of your wheelchair where no one else can see it. It holds about a gallon. The condom catheter nightmare, which empties into a bag attached to your calf with Velcro straps, holds about a quart of piss. If you're going to have something attached to you your whole life, it should at least be practical. Go for the options that suit your lifestyle. It takes forever to fill up a gallon bag, and when it is full, you can just tap a pal who's not squeamish and go out and empty the thing into a toilet or a drain or even on the side of the road, and Bob's your uncle (once more). It changed my life for the better, but my last weekend with a condom catheter was the turning point. It made me madder than a boot full of barbed wire. I'm surprised I still have teeth with all the grinding I did that night. But yes, something had to change, and this one incident made that paramount.

My wife went to the restaurant to meet more food reps, which is not half as fun as liquor reps, and it's already a moot decision, purely semantics. They are ahead of the booze reps. So she set me up on the pull-out couch in our living room back at the apartment because I was too tired (hungover) to go and wanted to catch up on a bit of sleep. I had a jug of water, some Valium, a down pillow, and what she would call mellow music loaded up in the cassette machine. Music choices are where we differ. The Who, The Stones, Elton John, and even April Wine are mellow music. Instead, she insisted on putting the Gypsy Kings into the cassette player, and "Oh well," she said, "you'll learn to like it, give it a chance. It's only a sixty-minute cassette, and then it turns off when it's over, so just suck it up and go with it." She was always trying to change my taste in music, and unfortunately, that did not happen (jazz still sucks ass). Somehow, she pressed repeat incessantly, going forwards and backward (it just kept rewinding), and I listened to eight life-sucking hours of the Gypsy Kings. Don't think I didn't try to "shut 'er down." I tried like hell, but the only thing I managed to do was pull on my condom catheter until I lost the whole rig. The sticky tape that goes around the shaft of my dick came right undone, and there was no draining into a bag. I pretty much just pissed like I was standing up, only I was laying down, and there was no way to stop from going piss. I couldn't just pinch my dick for eight hours. (I thought of it, but with my injury I can't squeeze anything.) I sure couldn't reattach the condom with my hands being pretty much useless. Damn you, opposable thumbs. So much for that pull-out mattress and so much for the Gypsy Kings. I would crawl over broken glass if it were to turn that shit off.

The mattress ended up in the trash bin (right next to the Gypsy Kings cassette), and I got an indwelling catheter a couple of days after that, "Nuff" said, except I want to kiss that guy from the Chinese restaurant. Things come to you one problem at a time, and with luck—and a little research— you try to solve them the best way you can. One gallon of piss beats a quart every time, and indwelling catheters rock, a sentence I thought would never come out of my mouth.

CHAPTER THIRTY-EIGHT

STEP FOUR: DEPRESSION

I'M GETTING AHEAD OF MYSELF. Before the Gypsy King marathon, we had to go through the process of hiring people to run the show. The booze choices came much later. I got ahead of myself because the booze choices were more kick-ass fun than the picking-the-staff choices. We rented a small community hall to interview potential waiters, cocktail waitresses, cooks, and whatever other randomly skilled, hard-working persons we could find that could help you build a pizza and sling a drink. You know how that went if you've ever hired people. Big ads in the newspaper, an extensive lineup of hopefuls waiting to give you a pumped-up, ten-page resume. The resumes become a blur. All I know is that everyone in that gym is highly overqualified to be working in a restaurant. My wife set up her little hiring table—complete with cardboard screens at one end, while my booth was across the gym a hundred feet away at the other end. We both read the identical resumes, complete with a reference marathon that went on and on about candidates that could have been canonized or sent straight to N.A.S.A.

There was a never-ending parade of people who wanted "a positive change" or wanted in on the "bottom floor." We had our own system all figured out. She would do an initial interview, dutifully reading every glowing resume, take notes, and send them to me, and then I would (supposedly) do the same thing. Later, the plan was to get together, compare notes over a couple of beers, and eliminate or call back the people we agreed were good candidates for the job. It was five hours of reading juiced-up life stories from people who wanted to be on our "Boston Pizza Team" (my wife's euphemism) and bring our franchise from fledgling status to roaring success. It soon became apparent that my wife read every resume and looked for diamonds in the rough: energetic, steady, hard-working types whom we could mold into greatness while I was hiring for Hooters. Fuck it. Who cared if they could even spell reference or qualification? If you look good, you get the job; we'll work out the details later. So chauvinistic, so non-pragmatic, so not what my wife was looking for. We did agree on a few people. I got to keep my blonde, smiling, generously endowed cocktail waitress and my savvy, world-weary but engaging bartender Bev, who was the most significant no-brainer hire of all.

She did the initial interview with my wife while I sat a hundred feet away, drinking my second 7-11 big gulp plastic cup filled with vodka and orange juice. I was a little pickled and apparently unaware of what was happening. I had gone outside about an hour earlier and emptied my leg bag (I was still doing the condom catheter at this point). Unfortunately, I had screwed up when it was time to return the clip to an upright position. Unbeknownst to me, I had been leaking piss all over the floor for the last hour. There was a healthy puddle underneath me and a stream flowing towards the double doors a hundred feet behind me as the floor slanted gently in that direction.

If I had looked, it was a blatantly obvious pond and stream combination, but I was bored and tapping a pencil singing a Boomtown Rat song in my head about not liking Mondays. Bev, whom I did not know at this point, stopped up short, about ten feet from me, and her facial expression said, "What the fuck." Shaking her head, she came toward me and, without a word, reached under the table I was sitting at and snapped my leg bag clip to the closed position. I looked around for a place to hide, realizing that I had been sitting in a pool of piss with two tributary streams for the last hour.

I smiled like a clown and said, "Thank you, and you're hired. How did you figure out that nightmare?"

She smiled, too, with a throaty half chuckle that invited you to laugh with her. "I have an aunt with the same rig. She's in a wheelchair and has the same forgetful problem you have," she informed me. "And I'm not cleaning that up," she added unnecessarily.

"I don't expect you to. And what are you applying for?"

"Bartender and I do have a resume."

"So what's it going to tell me? That you've always wanted to be a bartender and that it would be your dream job?"

"Fuck no. I mean, sure, I've been a bartender for six years and worked at some of the bigger hotels and nightclubs, but I'm going to school on Mondays and Wednesdays to be a hotel manager, so I'm not available on those days."

"Sold, or you're hired or whatever." I was happily drunk, and there was no one else in line, so I decided I would get to know my new bartender a little better. "So . . . nice tats," and she looked at me a little strange until my brain caught up to my mouth. "Uh, wait a minute, that came out all wrong. What do the tattoos represent, if you don't mind me asking? I'm kind of a tattoo guy." They were colorful and prominent, and you could tell from the get-go that she could care not a whit what you thought of them. They were the first semi-sleeve tattoos I'd ever seen.

"Which one?" She had a weird flower collage on her left arm with roses and other assorted flowers, with what looked like razor wire entwined around the bouquet, squeezing the shit out of it. The one on her right arm was a small heart and three names underneath it, with what looked like clouds and angels circling around, so I had to ask.

"Okay, I'll bite. Let's start with the heart arm. Whose names are those?"

"My younger siblings. My mother died young, and I helped raise them. She had me early, around seventeen, and kid number two popped out about twelve years later, followed by kid three and kid four in quick succession. And then she died, shitty timing."

"I'm sorry, that must have been hard." I felt an immediate comfort level with Bev, like I'd known her for years and this was some kind of weird high school reunion. We were just a couple of old friends catching up on the years we'd missed seeing each other. I was almost willing to share my big gulp, but there are limits.

"What are you sorry for?" she said dismissively. "She died a useless drunk with about ten dollars to her name, so nobody has to be sorry."

"I might have a small oral drug and alcohol addiction," I volunteered from nowhere. Bev chuckled again. It wasn't a laugh, more of a deep sound that said everything would be alright. I have a sense of humor that doesn't end, so laugh with me and I'll be your friend. She might have been thirty, maybe younger. She had one dimple and laugh lines around her eyes that seemed permanently fixed, white-blonde hair that might have been doctored (I wasn't about to ask), and she was tall and well built. I mean to say she had muscle definition in her arms and a bubble butt that just invited you to look at it, and she caught me red-handed doing that very thing when she stood up and adjusted her chair so her shoes were clear of the puddle of piss.

"Well, I think you could probably manage a hotel already, and I'm sure you can manage a Boston Pizza bar. So I'm going to hire you without looking at your credentials unless there's anything I need to know?"

"I've lived in Airdrie my whole life, and too late, I already saw you looking at my credentials. I can pour drinks faster than you can drink them, I'm good at handling drunk people, and I've never been to prison. Anything else you need to know?"

"Nope, all works for me, and I haven't been to prison lately either, but just a small heads up. I might be the drunkest guy in the room at any given time. Oh, and I'll be taking you up on your challenge about pourin' 'em faster than you can drink 'em, or I can drink 'em. I can drink 'em pretty fast," I slurred that last part. "We'll go from there. See you Saturday, it's the start of the training week, and I think we're all good from there."

"See you Saturday then," and I had hired a bartender. I wasn't sure what my wife thought of her, and I didn't care. On the other hand, I had a good feeling about her, and I had to know why she had a flower garden with razor wire wrapped around it tattooed forever on her left arm.

The rest of the afternoon drifted by in a drunken haze. People dropped by sporadically. I hired a couple of cooks that "looked" efficient and the dishwasher since only one applied. My wife picked the rest after we sat down and compared notes. She even phoned the references provided. I mean, really? Who puts down a reference from their parole officer or the last boss that turfed them out the door. Actually, you'd be surprised, but finally, we had our staff, thirty or so people who were going to get our franchise off the ground.

I'll spare you all the details, give or take, because it's relentlessly boring watching training videos and teaching people how to make the dough, weigh ingredients, and say "order in." My Hooters chick named Tammy (or Tammy the waitress, as I later call her) was a surprise. She could charm you out of your wallet and your credit cards and make you feel good about it, while Bev served up the overpriced drinks at a pace of a hardened veteran—and no, I couldn't drink that fast. That would come later. It was fun to watch, and watch I did. Between the kitchen and the bar was a swinging door that only swung one way for me after a hard day of training the newbies. Luckily, Boston Pizza dispatched a crew to every new opening to do the "training thing" anyway, so my participation was relegated to a few tips from experiences I had already learned. Nods of approval mixed in with a few exasperated, "What the fuck are you thinking? You forgot to put cheese on that, and it's a *pizza*. For God's sake, all pizzas get cheese. Who the fuck ever ate a pizza without cheese?" You know, small tips that make you a better pizza cooker until my wife looked exasperated. Then it was off to, and through, the swinging doors.

I thought I was a pretty good boss and communicated well with lots of laughs and lots of fuckups—or learning experiences, as I like to call them. They sure figured out quickly that when they screwed up a pizza, they had to eat the mistake, a perk that came about far too often. It did help a pantload that the head office kitchen trainer they sent in from Richmond, B.C. just happened to be my good friend Scott Adams, and we had already done this dance more than once. It went smoothly, but I found myself sneaking out the swinging doors earlier each night and sitting at the end of the bar in my spot. The first rule about owning a restaurant was that you didn't have to pay for drinks. So right about seven each evening, there would be a smiling Bev holding out a triple Gibson's (three onions, not olives) slightly dry martini, made with Tanqueray gin. At the same time, Tammy the waitress, the "sweater girl," smiled and flipped through the local paper as she sat cross-legged on a barstool. She couldn't reach the bottom rail as she stood about five feet nothing. Tammy the waitress was like a miniature California Barbie if Barbie was more well-endowed. She had pouty lips you wanted to kiss and eyes you could lose yourself in, unblemished fake-tan skin, and a how-do-you-do smile. She was clever, well-read, and could carry fifteen assorted glasses with a tray in one hand while she took your tips with the other. I deemed her and Bev "untrainable" once they learned how the cash register worked, and they were good to go, fully trained, and customer-friendly.

"Hi Bev, and thank you," I said on training day number six. We were getting a run-through tomorrow, where you give invitations to all the businesses in the neighborhood. Some you take to the police station or the fire station, a night of free food and introductions.

"No problem. What do you want me to put that under?" Bev asked needlessly. Luckily, free-pour drinks were never tabulated, while the friggin' shotgun, button-controlled shithouse liquor was on the record. So you had to account for every ounce of nasty, cheap house gin, vodka, rye, and rum, while the "primo" stuff just sat on the racks behind the bar screaming, "drink me," until it became obvious.

"Just put 'er under spillage, and my good friend Adams will be thirsty too. Bev . . . charge him double because he's got a company credit card. And buy the quiet one sitting on the barstool reading a newspaper a drink too, and yourself, of course."

"Yeah, I know. So keep spilling and billing, and keep them coming."

Best hire ever. Bev kept the drinks coming for about eleven days in a row, and Adams finally had to declare the restaurant officially open. I even got an extra five days out of him that was paid for by head office because I played the "Quad Card," my new superpower, which I kept pretty close to my chest.

Adams's expense account was a bonus, and we kicked the living shit out of that account. He got busted on that one. He went way over his limit, but he played *my* "Quad Card" too, so what could they do?

Yep, that's pretty much how it went, the "Hi, Bev" was happening earlier each day, but I did hire some pleasant surprises. I had a decent kitchen manager, Jason, and a couple of all-star cooks, Murray and Curtis. And of course, Michelle, the one in the background who kept bins filled with ingredients and made pizza dough when necessary. If I were walking, she's the one that would have challenged my ability to say, "No, I'm a married man." Boy, earlier on, I heavily sucked at being hitched, but so did my wife. We were so intent on opening our restaurant that we had neglected our marriage. We went to bed too tired to do anything but talk briefly about the restaurant. I was getting restauranted out. My condition was not to be discussed. It was as if Quadriplegia was sidelined if it wasn't mentioned outright. Home support got me up every morning. I sat on the commode three times a week, got dressed, and rushed right back to the restaurant to soldier on.

Every day I would powerchair to the restaurant around eleven. We lived only three and a half blocks away over a tiny bridge. It was a bridge that went over a small creek, and it had a hell of a slope that tested my wheelchair driving skills daily. But some things did get easier. Thankfully, home support was no longer a problem. A beautiful (inside and out) pint-sized Portuguese woman—I had sent the weird mothball lady packing—was fantastic. Marie, a little slip of a woman with a huge heart. A woman who mothered me. She scolded me, and yet she made me feel good about myself. She stuck a finger up my butt inserting suppositories, and she let me sit in the shower on the bath seat for as long as I wanted. Man, there is something about a shower with unlimited hot water and excellent water pressure. My aches and pains sluiced down the drain.

Unfortunately, it was still not ideal to be a drunk Quad. Only one invariably was related to the other. Driving home was always an adventure. I had traded one addiction for another. Demerol was off the table, but Amitriptyline and Valium, along with Baclofen and Gabapentin, were my constant companions. The results of such abuse were a done deal. Something had to give. One day I was going home around eight or eight-thirty in minus seventeen-degree weather, and I forgot about the slope on the damn bridge. More importantly, I didn't lean forward. I was probably leaning four different ways at that point, but leaning backward was the wrong way to bend, and my dozen-plus martinis might have contributed to the problem. Old Bert, the powerchair, flipped back (fuck you wheelie bars, they're for wimps) and had me looking at the stars halfway up the ridiculous tiny bridge, named appropriately later as the "brain-buster" bridge. It was essentially a small bridge in a small park, so nobody I knew was going to happen by, and random strangers coming through the park at this late hour were about as likely as me getting up and walking the rest of the way. I could tell my head was bleeding again. I put my hand above my head where my baseball hat had not done its secondary job as a pseudo helmet, and my hand came back all sticky and dark. Just another stinkin' head wound. Still, I could deal with that, business as usual.

It was a clear night. I lay there stargazing, and I thought of my friend Larry, or Lar (rhymes with bar), as his friends called him, who came to the grand opening. He was from my hometown, Maple Ridge. We were strolling back to the apartment from the restaurant as opening day happened in the middle of a cold snap. We were with family members and friends who had also made the trip. The temperature had dropped to minus twenty-five (minus thirteen in Fahrenheit), and Lar vehemently postulated, "You are one stupid son of a bitch if you think there are different kinds of cold. Fuck the humidity factor; this is cold. Stupid people who think a dry cold is different than a wet cold are fucked in the head. It's pure bullshit. Cold is cold."

Well, I lay there, just me and my busted brain on the upslope of the bridge, feeling a tingle in my thumbs as they headed for frostbite; I considered Lar a brilliant man. Cold is fucking cold, wet or dry.

My wife used this bridge to get home at times. Still, she stayed later each night to unwind and play darts with after-hour customers, so I lay there for what seemed like hours. Once the booze wore off, I started shivering. Every muscle was tense, my shoulders were shaking involuntarily, and my teeth were clacking together like tiny castanets. I tried hard to picture myself sitting in that stinging hot shower.

I was also thinking, "what a piss-poor place to die"; I survived twenty-two car accidents and three motorcycle accidents (I was the worst driver on the planet), and this is where it all ends, on a goddamn bridge that spans a little frozen creek. I was feeling sorry for myself that night, melancholy, useless. I was content just to lay there. I didn't call for help, resigned to my fate, and was almost relieved. Bring it on. I'm ready.

I was strangely disappointed when this did not happen. Marie, scheduled to put me to bed at ten that night, was searching for me (bless her heart), mostly because I had drunkenly blown off all time constraints and was an ass for not calling ahead. Usually, I would call Marie and tell her when I knew I would be late or early, and she was nice enough to work around my inability to be responsible. Fortunately, Marie lived two blocks away, and when I wasn't home by ten, the search was on. Two hours later, when she found me, I was shivering my ass off and barely conscious. She somehow got me lifted back upright (I think she went straight to the restaurant and brought some burly men with her). Still, somehow I woke up in bed several hours later, sketchy on the details, covered with three blankets and two hot water bottles that were stuffed under my arms. I had a soft spot on my head that was almost a squishy bruise and a broken baby finger that was of little consequence. I should have removed the damn things because I had no feeling in those little fingers anyway, and they always got caught in the wheels or some other part of the chair. That would not be the last time I looked up at the night sky, counting stars, real or imagined, with broken fingers. It was a portent of things to come, but at least *this* time I incurred no permanent damage. Hurray, three cheers for whoever forgives fools and drunks, because I qualified on both counts. I just couldn't shake that nagging feeling of disappointment that someone had found me before I froze to death.

CHAPTER THIRTY-NINE

MORE DEPRESSION, NAGGING DEPRESSION

I THINK YOU GET THE gist of what became my normal. First, I learned lessons the hard way. I learned not to lean back in the chair, especially not on the brain-buster bridge. I realized that dry cold and humid cold were not different, especially when you're on your back on a bridge and your head is bleeding. Second, I did not blame the booze. I've said this more than once, like an addict's lament. If I blamed the alcohol, I might have to cut down on my daily limit, which seemed unlikely. If spillage became a big thing (my money partners were nitpicky assholes at times), I would change the game plan. I would bring my giant wineskin—the perfect smuggler size for concerts and hockey games, thirty ounces—and I would fill it with complimentary wine (gotta love booze reps). I would go cruising, just me and old Bert hitting the trails and the highways, *chug-a-lug, chug-a-lug*, and this was not always a good thing. I would eventually end up back at the restaurant, where I was quickly turning into just an underpaid flunky—a drunky flunky. I chimed in now and then with pizza restaurant platitudes which, in my drunken mind, made me think I was still managing the back half of the restaurant.

"Remember, people, pizza first, then pasta. Pasta is just reheated al dente noodles and a scoop of secret sauce. Time to make a batch of pizza dough. Quit eating all the products, Jason. Don't they feed you at home?" And that was my contribution. The restaurant has been managed. Good job, Randy, well done. You deserve a due diligence drink.

"Oh, and take over for me, you overworked, underpaid motherfuckers, because I'll be in the bar, through those swing doors, if anyone needs me. And what the fuck, if you get hungry, feel free to fuck up a pizza order or two; just bring me the bill." So yessiree, the job is done. Now it's time to manage *myself*, which required little effort and did not advance my station in life. My life meant nothing; I was a drag on the system, sand in the gears. I drank like a Viking and took drugs in amounts that would have killed a crack addict, and I felt I was losing control of my mind, identity, life, and wife. I was disappearing as the months passed. Finally, summer rolled around, and my self-destructive behavior wasn't getting any better. If anything, it was getting worse.

I would hold my arm up sometimes and imagine I could look right through it because I was turning fucking invisible, but I would still gamely motor on—just me, Bert, and my wineskin. Nobody gave a shit if I was there or not.

The afternoon started as it usually did. Bev was filling 'em up as fast as I could drink 'em down. Gin and pickled onions being my drink of choice that day, it rarely changed. Bev was my new best friend—a captive friend, to be sure—but we chatted for hours and exchanged stories, good and bad. She could easily use both the right and the left sides of her brain. By this time, being a drunk was almost a daily necessity. I didn't even pretend to work at the restaurant. My wife and I were strangers, and believe me, she had every reason to be disgusted. However, it wasn't the restaurant or the things I could still control that set the wheels in motion. It was a fuckhead drunk asshole that chose to sit at the bar that afternoon. I had seen and dismissed him a handful of times. "Fuck it," I told Bev more than once. "He's drinking and paying, and he brings his buddies most times who also drink and pay, so just ignore the asshole. No worries."

But this one afternoon, he brought no drinking buddies with him, and he showed up drunk. Then he invaded my space, perched himself on a barstool, and insulted Bev and Tammy the waitress. He was a mere ten feet away, and I could hear every rude, stupid comment. All I could think of was how much I hated the rude and stupid. I was staring at him, unaware I was doing so.

"What are you looking at, wheelchair clown?" he asked because he noticed me staring at him, or "gunning him," as my old friend Jimmy Franklin would say. So many fights started back in my hometown if you found somebody gunning you.

Bev could see me gritting my teeth and steaming, but she came around behind me, went straight up to him, grabbed his elbow, and calmly escorted him to a four-top in the far corner of the bar, handling the situation efficiently. She came back and shrugged it off.

"What are you going to do? People are assholes," she said calmly, but her hands were shaking slightly, which was strange for Bev, who was not only a great bartender but could have moonlighted as a bouncer.

"Yeah, Bev, believe me, I know, but I still think rude sucks. I hate rude fucking people, and I hate them that much more since I've been in this fucking chair. Sorry you had to deal with that shit."

"Yeah, asshole drunks are the same the world over, but that one obviously bothered you more than most. It's like your eyes got all black and shit. You looked kinda scary." Maybe my hands were shaking too, and I felt strangely protective. She got me another martini, and I tried to forget about the drunk asshole, but Bev could sense it was still on my brain, so she switched tracks on me. "You know," she said, "it's funny that you never did ask about the rose garden tattoo. I got that one for a marriage I had, and a second one that was a marriage I royally screwed up."

"Huh, say what? And that's a seven martini 'say what,' because I have no idea what you're talking about. You just jumped tracks; good deflection technique."

"Well, you asked about my heart tattoo during my job interview, and you never did ask about the other one."

"I'll bite. What's with the rose garden tattoo?" She was good. I almost forgot about the asshole.

"Okay, it's two tattoos in one. It's all about my first husband, and it got an add-on after I got married again. I should've learned after the first one."

"Tell me about the first one."

"Think about it. The first marriage happens with all the trimmings. You're naïve and hopeful. You pick out an expensive wedding dress with three or four of your best friends or relatives, and out of that group, you have to pick a maid of honor without pissing off your close friends who didn't get picked. You rent a hall, hire a band, buy a shit-ton of booze, and get drunk. Finally, the wedding cake gets handed out, and you're left twisting in the wind, seventeen years old with zero survival skills."

"You just described my mother's wedding. Seventeen is a little young."

"Okay, it's a little young, I agree, but my first husband was like a demo version of a husband. I think I was just trying it on to see how it fit. He was sparkly and clean."

"I can say I've never heard it put quite that way. So . . . you drove the Pinto demo and then traded up to the next husband. Pinto to Cadillac?"

"No, let me finish. The first guy was the Cadillac. I was just too stupid to know it. He didn't party his ass off. He was polite, attentive, understanding, and boring as all get-out. He did, however, think my friends were total fuck-ups, and that I drank too much, stayed out way too late, and generally did not give a shit. In the end, he was right. A lot of my friends were total fuck-ups. I drank a shit-ton and came home whenever I wanted to. I just wasn't ready to change my life at that point, so I snorted cocaine on toilet tanks in about a dozen bathrooms, danced on the edge of the cliff, and partied all night long."

"This sounds vaguely familiar," I said as she continued mixing drinks without breaking stride, and I kept looking across the bar as I thought of one hundred ways to kill a drunk asshole with my wheelchair. Unfortunately, I had a one-track mind, and it was hard to switch off, although Bev was still trying.

"Okay, so the story of the tattoo. Back to the first guy I married. He was gold. We got along great; he had a heart as big as all outdoors and would do anything for me. He would have jumped in front of a train for me. So anyway, we went to the Calgary Stampede one day, and I won a mechanical bull-riding contest."

"Will wonders never cease." I was still listening, picturing Bev riding a mechanical bull, and it was not a bad picture.

"Fuck off, so the prize for staying on the bull was two hundred bucks, so I got a belt buckle and this tattoo. This tattoo is where my prize money went . . . well, and a little more," and Bev rolled up her sleeve for emphasis. "The first husband wanted a rose garden tattoo, so I went with it. He said this way he would never have to buy me roses, all I had to do was look at my arm and I would think of him. He actually said that as I was getting the tattoo."

"Okay, that is so fucking corny I want to puke. So, what happened to the guy? The Cadillac, the trial guy, whatever? How did you fuck that up?" She had piqued my interest.

"Don't give me that look. Everyone seems to screw up the first marriage. At least in my experience. It's kind of a rite of passage. I eventually cheated on husband number one, the Cadillac. I took him for granted and kicked him out the door before he kicked me out. He rebounded, found his prom queen three years later, two kids, and a large house payment, none of the shit that excited me at that time of my life. In the end, he got what he was looking for, and we got divorced. I don't expect a redo or anything, but it makes me think, what if?"

"So . . . ?"

"Yeah, yeah, the razor wire is for another day."

"Somehow, I think I'm supposed to get something out of that story. It's like an *Aesop's Fable* thingy, isn't it, and there's a lesson or a moral I'm supposed to pick up on?"

"Yeah, I'm not very subtle, and you're fucking stupid. But damn right, you're supposed to get something out of it. I don't know who in hell Aesop is. I'm just looking at *your* marriage. You two seem more like strangers every day, if that makes any sense, but you can't see it because you're too close to it."

"Okay, now you're pissing me off. Let's stick with your marriage. Mine is currently off the table. So what's with the fuckin' razor wire?"

"Well, I mean, isn't it obvious? It's not razor wire, it's supposed to be barbed wire, and it's choking the shit out of my roses. It represents, no . . . it *reminds* me of the guy I cheated with, who screwed up my first marriage. He's the personification of the barbed wire. The second guy I eventually married because I'm an idiot. He's the guy that follows me around, and I will never shake until I leave Airdrie in the rear-view mirror."

"Okay, so go out and get a restraining order or a divorce or something. Airdrie is small, but you can still avoid him, get a new boyfriend, some-body big and ugly, start hanging out somewhere else, change your job, change your life . . . Oh shit, I think I just got it. Really? What the fuck?"

"You got there on your own. I'm impressed after all the booze you consume regularly."

"Booze sometimes gives me clarity. I get a revelation now and then. So, the guy that fucked up your marriage, the guy you eventually married, the fucking Pinto, is the asshole sitting right over there?"

"His name is Brian, and you are so right. He is an asshole."

"Go tell him to leave. Tell him I'll pick up his tab, and he can fuck right off. I'll be your restraining order."

"Yeah, I've been thinking about that. Cut Brian the asshole off before he becomes a bigger problem, but *I'll* take care of the tab," and Bev did that very thing. She could be a take-no-prisoners hard ass when she wanted to be. He argued his case weakly, but he got up and made his way to the door. Unfortunately, he flips the finger, guns me, and gets in the last word as he walks out.

"So they have to 'Bring out the gimp.' I'll be back, you little cock-biter," and I was so surprised that he had watched *Pulp Fiction*, I had no snappy comeback. Then, of course, I thought of about twenty when he was gone, George Costanza style, but I put the whole thing on hold for the health of my brain and well-being and ordered a shooter for Tammy the waitress and Bev and of course myself. I wasn't good at drinking alone, and I felt like drinking more than usual.

"So, back to *your* marriage," she said after polishing off a three-ounce shooter of Bailey's and vodka.

"Are we talking about Wagner's marriage?" says Tammy the waitress, who has wandered into my space, and she orders another shooter and puts her arm around my shoulder. "It's about time. It's not like we haven't talked about it a hundred times when you aren't here." Apparently I don't have a "my space."

"Fuck that, that is for another day, my marriage is off-limits, especially for bartenders and waitresses, but I will take another martini and a beer for everyone in the kitchen. It sounds like a good finish to the day. Fuck marriage talk." So I bought the kitchen staff three pitchers of beer, and I suggested they drink it out of coffee cups because even though it was a slow night, I'm not sure my wife would have sanctioned that gesture. But I was proven wrong shortly afterward, as she dropped by the bar, ran the restaurant from the stool at the bar, and drank shooters with the crew. Damn, she was efficient.

After two more shooters and two more martinis, I should have just gone home, but instead I bought the kitchen staff two more pitchers of beer, and I lost control of my environment. It was no big deal. It cost me nothing and made me look like a hero. The restaurant wasn't killer busy, and the kitchen staff was mainly legal because eighteen was the drinking age in Alberta. I never once thought about how a drunk kitchen staff might perform. That wasn't my job. My job was morale, and I was rocking my job.

"Do you watch the news?" Bev asked after the asshole went home. She had personally escorted him out and she now hanging around my spot, like everyone else. Bev was filling the odd drink order, as there were still six or seven stragglers hanging around. Tammy the waitress had participated in the six ounces of the instant shooter buzz, but she could handle the stragglers, so why not run with it? Yup, I had lost control. Tammy the waitress, my wife, and Bev shared a jug of margaritas filed under just another mistake. It was a big-time mistake day. Even my wife was participating because a drunk restaurant is a happy restaurant. She was sitting in the bar and drinking like a trooper on leave by that time. It was good to see her relax.

"Okay, yeah, I watch the news," I offered up, still listening after Bev had asked the question. "I wanted to be Tony Parsons when I grew up. He always looked so unflappable."

"Whoever the hell he is, old man; I don't know which news you watch. But I'm talking about the guy who got hit by lightning, which has nothing to do with Tony Parsons. Did you see that? The lightning guy?"

"Nope, I missed that one," I replied. Bev had the floor. We all kind of forgot we had customers.

"Okay, this guy was in a wheelchair, like you or kind of like you. Anyway, he's going home one day in a storm and gets hit by lightning, like full-on. He gets all fucked up like he's electrocuted, but he lives. I think it blew him right out of his shoes."

"Okay, so where are we going with this?" I'm trying to think of Tony Parsons getting hit by lightning, but I think I'll shelf Tony for now. He'd probably just shrug it off and keep on informing the public.

"Let me finish, no hijacking. So this guy gets hit by lightning and is rushed to the hospital. The next thing you know, he can feel his legs, and he was paralyzed before he got zapped, so he lies in the hospital for a while, and the feeling in his legs starts coming back. I mean, he's not like walking and shit, but he can feel his toes and he can stand up with just a little help."

"I call bullshit," I say with conviction. "That just can't happen. Your spinal cord can't spontaneously heal because you get lightninged, if that's a word."

"Hey," says Bev, "I'm just telling you what I watched."

So now Tammy the waitress chirps up. "C'mon, that just makes sense. So, like, your whole body is dependent on electrical impulses, and isn't lightning, like, electric?"

"Thanks, Doctor Tammy, I'll consider that," says my wife as she joins in with a nod and an expective look. I'm now talking to fools, and all three of them are looking at the biggest one of them.

"I guess it can't hurt to try," I say, but I'm skeptical. The news these two watch is more like that stupid *Believe It Or Not* television show. This is an old wives' tale in the making. But I'm a gamer. "So you're suggesting I go out and get hit by lightning? You can't be serious?"

Bev holds up her hands and gives everyone another round of shooters. The spillage is getting huge. I have an extremely clumsy staff. Who hired these people? The last customer has left the bar, and I closed it down early, so now we're all sitting around drinking, and Tammy the waitress will not let it go.

"I only mention it," she says, "because there is supposed to be a big storm tonight, and what have you got to lose?"

Now I'm looking around. My wife, Tammy the waitress, Bev, and the kitchen manager, who has also joined us, all nod in unison. This idea is starting to get legs. So we all discuss it over a few more drinks. I don't know who the fuck is running the restaurant, but I am not worried about that. Dishes can wait. I'm more concerned about this crazy idea forming in my head, and after a few more drinks, I voice my opinion. I am considering being a big-ass lightning rod.

"You're all suggesting that I should get hit by lightning. You guys are all thinking about it, I can tell, and maybe you're right. What have I got to lose? Lightning could be my new best friend," but I realize how fucked up that sounds after I say it.

"Uh . . . you could die," says Tammy the waitress, but she's holding up her hands like she's juggling the idea, and everyone else is juggling this idea in their minds. There's a pregnant silence that stretches on for another couple of seconds as the whole crowd is juggling, and I finally relent to the inevitable. I have reached that point where I'm slurring every second word.

"Ah, fuck it then, damn the shorpedoes, letch give this shit a real try, but if we're going to do this, letch ramp up the odds. I should hold up a golf club or shomething."

"You know what," says the kitchen manager, who generally has no opinion about anything, "we should wrap you in tinfoil. That way, you attract lightning. Tinfoil is like the next best thing to a lightning rod."

I'm fully engaged by now, and I'm going along with this story. "Yup, it is, so letch gets it on. The storm is right here. Why waste a good storm?" I realize we are *all* fucking loopy drunk, and the next thing that happens is inevitable. I'm not sure if my wife is looking for renewed feeling in my legs or the instant death that might occur if lightning strikes me, but after a couple more shooters and some Giant Mugs of beer, it seemed like a good idea to someone above my pay grade. Giant Mugs, sometimes referred to as Thunder Mugs, were the new promotional gimmick, a Boston Pizza special that was all fucked up. Head office brought in cases of these twenty-four-ounce mugs that weighed about five pounds, and everyone just stole the damn things.

I think I might have had three of those Giant Mugs to finish my drunken pursuits. I lost count as the party was in full swing, and the next thing you know, we're all in the kitchen wrapping me in tinfoil. It's a gang-up, a dog-pile. I slightly protest, but it falls on deaf ears. Everyone is chirping about the chances of me getting hit by lightning, and Tammy the wait-ress suggests that conductivity is the key, and they're all fucking laughing. I'm treating it like a team-building exercise. I don't know where the hell Tammy the waitress suddenly got all lightning savvy, but off she goes to the parking lot while they are wrapping me in tinfoil, and she suddenly appears with a hubcap. An honest-to-goodness Lincoln Town car hubcap. The fucking thing is more than a foot and a half in diameter—it looks like a Vietnamese rice-picking hat—and she wants to put it on my head. I know this is fucked up beyond reason, but we're all laughing our asses off, and the kitchen manager has gone to get duct tape. If you're going to get dressed in a tinfoil suit and wear a hubcap on your head, duct tape is necessary. It turns into a feat of drunken engineering. I am a captive and participatory audience. Even the line cooks and some of the front-end waitresses have come to witness this crazy escapade.

Almost the entire staff is involved as duct tape is applied. My cred-ibility as a manager is going up in smoke, and I'm starting to look like a tinfoil mummy. The foil is tucked in all around me. It won't impede my progress and get caught in the wheels, and they all step back to look at their handiwork.

The hubcap is somehow duct-taped securely to my head, and I feel like fucking *Don Quixote*. I am a man with a mission, tilting at forked lightning instead of windmills. The next step is to find some high ground and get struck by lightning. After that, we all have another shooter. My tinfoil suit crinkles away as I slam down a giant tequila. Everyone decides in the end that this is a singular mission. The rain is coming down in buckets, and only an idiot (I can hear my mother's voice) would go out in this storm. I am escorted to the restaurant's back door to the wheelchair ramp with my cheerleader crowd. Someone hands me a car aerial, presumably ripped off a car in the parking lot, probably the Lincoln (no one could find a golf club). Everyone is laughing, and there is a collective cheer as off I go into the rain and the storm. You can hear the thunder in the distance, and you can see the black clouds rolling over the Rockies that are coming my way. It's raining hard.

I decided I would go straight to the brain-buster bridge, and there I sat, shitfaced, still sipping on my half-filled wineskin, my constant companion.

I wonder who filled that up? I'm holding up a car aerial with a fucking hubcap on my head, all wrapped up in tinfoil. At first, I yelled unintelligible challenges to some obscure lightning god, but I quieted as time wore on. I was the only one out there, and weirdly enough, I secretly wanted to get hit by lightning. Getting some more feeling in my body seemed like a no-brainer in my inebriated mind. I considered no other downfalls, although I could hear my friend Mike Bignell in my ear. He was not the author of the saying, "Nothing good can come of this," but it carried weight when he did say it. I believe I sat there for close to two hours, slipping in and out of consciousness, the driving rain playing staccato on the foil. It's hard to pass out when there is a tambourine of unrelenting rain on tinfoil.

There was even a smattering of hail to change the mood, and little ice balls are always angry. I wondered if it could puncture my tin foil suit. I semi-consciously watched as the storm came and went, and I'm sure I would have been committed to the psych ward if anyone had seen me as I sat there stoically, patiently waiting for the big jolt. All I got was a shiver I couldn't control and an earful of the driving rain deflecting off my hubcap and my tinfoil costume. The lightning had passed miles to the north of me. I was severely disappointed, but the rain wasn't going anywhere. If anything, it was coming down harder. I sat there, going in and out of awareness, until I felt a light touch on my shoulder. For a minute, I almost forgot where I was. It always amazes me how a dozen shooters can come up and grab your ass.

"Okay, thunder god, I think the storm didn't *pick* you, and it's time to find your way back home." I know that voice, my little reptilian voice chirps up in my head.

"What the fuck are you doing here? You could have been electrocuted or worse. You don't even have an umbrella. That's a fucking bad move in a lightning storm. So, you didn't happen to pack a Gibson martini with pickled onions with you?"

"That's your go-to. The guy wrapped in tin foil and wearing a hubcap tells me I could get electrocuted. But no, I think we're done with me serving you martinis, and it looks like you're half frozen, so let's go. Better luck next time. If you do something like this again, I want no part of it."

I eventually, somehow, steered Bert back to the apartment. Back to the stable like a runaway horse. I magically arrived there, and Marie was still there. Unfortunately, I had forgotten to call her again, but in my mind she seemed unperturbed. She acted like she expected me. I had failed to care about such things at this point. "It's real late. So what the fuck? Why are you here?"

"Your wife called me."

"Are you nuts? It's like one o'clock in the morning."

"It's only a little after midnight, and I worry about you. I am not just your home support worker. I am your friend, and I see unhappiness in you. I toilet you, shower you, and put the clothes on you every morning, and you never smile. It is like someone has taken your smile. Where I come from, people smile in the best of times, and they smile harder at the worst of times."

"You realizsh yer talkin' to a human man with a hubbacap on his head, wrapped in a hundered, hundered yards o' tinfoil. If that ain't funny, what is?" I think I was laughing it off, but I can only remember little snippets for the life of me.

"Yes, and that is the problem. You are willing to let people laugh at you, but you don't laugh back." I think that was Marie, or maybe not, it was too deep for Marie.

That sobered me slightly. "What are you, a fucking Portgoose psychologist? I don't need someone dissecting my fucking life," and I regretted it as soon as I said it. From what I remember, she never said another word, and I was unwrapped, like a giant practical joke Christmas present that nobody wants. I felt so bad, and it was hard not to puke. I should have never been an asshole to Marie, someone who wanted to take care of me and who worried about me and my headspace. I was being a dickhead. Finally, the wrapping paper came off, and I had a new healthy respect for duct tape. That shit is impressive. *Red Green* was right. It could do anything, but a lot of hair comes with it when you take it off. Chunks of my hair were cut out, someone pulled and someone cut, and there was no alternative; the stuff is worse than gum.

I imagine I would have whined if I wasn't drunk beyond pain, and I passed out even as my hair was being cut. Every time I tried to fall asleep over my legs, I was picked up and held steady as my hair was abused. Marie then talked to me. It felt like she was talking to someone else because I was close to comatose, but I got instructions not to go to the restaurant tomorrow, and someone made me a large cup of green tea and sat and watched me as I spasmed like crazy and tried to get some warmth back in my bones. I hated myself. This wonderful five-foot beautiful Portuguese woman was the only one who cared for me, and I had disappointed her. I had taken her for granted. It was all about me, and I was ruining the one good thing in my life by beaking my mouth off like a spoiled child. I didn't know what to say to make everything all right again. I drank my tea and tried to focus, as I was still drunk twice over, and I didn't even realize I was crying until she came up and wiped my face with a Kleenex. I think she was silently crying too, and we both laughed a little in the end. "You're cut off," was the last thing I remember before getting my comatose ass into bed.

I woke up at nine the following day with Marie shaking me. We didn't talk about the night before, which was a good thing. I remembered very little of what had happened, drunken black spots, total voids in my memory, like how I even made it home. I did wonder, however, where my wife was. Marie explained that she had phoned her and told her she was staying at a friend's place because she was too drunk to drive. Too drunk to drive, even though we lived four blocks away.

CHAPTER FORTY

NOT DEPRESSION, MORE LIKE CONFUSION, NOT A STEP

THREE HUNDRED AND THIRTY-FIVE DAYS. One month away from being in a wheelchair for almost a year. Still no sparing, still no tingling. I had pretty much given up on getting hit by proverbial lightning. Although that felt like a lifetime ago, it had only been a week. It seems I had peaked as far as getting any more feeling back, and I had been wearing my Boston Pizza baseball cap since that night. I vaguely remember getting my hair cut, but you can't fool a mirror. It looked like a third grader had scored their first pair of scissors and made me into an art project.

The kitchen staff gave me a thumbs up every morning or afternoon that I showed up at the restaurant, and I got the odd backslap like I was one of the guys. My credibility was low, and I was no longer a manager, but I somehow managed to get an inventory done every month. I wrote down staff hours, scheduled them accordingly, and ordered the required product without messing it up. I was good at *that* part. I had an organized brain, and somewhere back in my juiced brain, I wanted the goddamn restaurant to do well.

It was a week after the day I didn't get hit by lightning. I was taking up space at the end of the bar right outside the double swinging doors when Bev called me an idiot. She wasn't big on rolling me out the door into the storm and regretted letting me power merrily away covered in tinfoil. Tammy the waitress was still laughing, but she would have laughed through the sinking of the Titanic. There is no regret in Tammy the waitress. I tried to give her the hubcap back, but I was informed that she had no idea which car it came off of; she didn't care that there was a Lincoln Town car without a hubcap and quite possibly an aerial. So I set it up behind the bar like a souvenir to remind me what a doofus I was. It was less important than the signed jerseys from the Edmonton Oilers and the Vancouver Canucks, and an autographed stick from Al MacInnis—thank you, Adams. These were the showcase items in the sports bar, and now I had a hubcap—my very own "showcase" item. Naturally, Bev didn't like it.

"C'mon, Bev. You were standing there wrapping me in tin foil too. Let's just call it a *thing* and get on with our little lives." It was a weird day. I felt a little melancholy, and the booze crushed my inhibitions. "Your asshole boyfriend pissed me off more than you could know, and I needed a distraction."

"You call him my boyfriend one more time, and I will force-feed you ground glass until you slowly die," and the smile ran away from her face. I think that's in a Billy Joel song.

"Okay, okay, sorry. Your sort-of-ex-husband, your stalker, whatever, but it did fuck me up."

"Why would that be a big deal? I tell you about my mother and how I raised my siblings, and you key in on the stupid tattoo and the ex-husband, the one I have erased from my memory. Your self-importance pisses me off. What's that got to do with you?"

"Yeah, okay, I'll give you that. Why are you so touchy? Wait till you end up in a wheelchair. Then you can't help thinking about it. You can't un-think about it. You do get self-absorbed and, yeah, self-important. You start relating everything around you to your predicament. Are there stairs? Is there a bed I can transfer into at the end of the night? Oh and wait, don't stop there. My favorite, did I have a good routine, or will I suddenly have that five-minute feeling where I must find a fucking toilet before I shit myself? Yeah, I worry about that. I'm sure your siblings are fine, especially if they turned out like you."

"One is a dead shithead, one is in Ontario and doesn't talk to me, and one is living with me while he finishes his course in nursing. Thanks for asking."

"Yeah, okay, I should have asked. Why won't one talk to you?""

"I picked an asshole on the second go-round. She disapproved of him. But unfortunately, she attached herself to that piece of shit. So now she talks to my ex-husband. She considers him the one that got screwed in the end." She tells me this as her voice rises. We're both a little louder than usual.

"I don't get it either. He's an instant asshole, and you can tell that from the get-go. Reading people is not my strong point, but that was as obvious as a good kick in the nuts. Maybe that's why my best friends are all the ones I grew up with, and I never had to choose one over the other or try to figure out what they were thinking or what they would do next. I just knew, and I didn't have to do any people reading."

"What's to fucking get? I'm a self-destructive screw-up. I make bad choices. I looked it up once, and there are all types of relationships. My husband was codependent. He couldn't exist without me, which was suffocating. It smothered me. He couldn't do a single fucking thing without me. I'm not going to bore you with the other types, just that I was into toxic relationships, where everything is a fight, a challenge, and the only good sex was make-up sex. We both did whatever the fuck we wanted to, and at the end of the day, we still had each other no matter how many times we threatened to kill each other."

"You're right. That's pretty fucked up. I could've done without hearing that last bit," I muttered to myself.

"Yeah, well, I outgrew it. It became unhealthy. But still, the asshole is just making it more difficult, if not impossible. Brian turns up everywhere, knocking on my door drunk, coming to my work, calling me at all hours until I have to answer or just turn my goddamn phone off."

"Tell him you're in another relationship, that there's no hope for him, and to fuck right off." And then there was this strange, uncomfortable silence, a little void had crept in on silent feet, not something Bev nor I ever experienced before. We both started looking around at other stuff, just not at each other. She had a weird apologetic look on her face, she cleared her throat a couple of times, and then a stray tear came out of nowhere. "What?" I said as I'm not really good with emotions. I don't hug anything out in my dealings with people, and I don't lick stray tears off anyone's face, although weirdly enough, that thought flitted by. Still, I couldn't help thinking I was missing something. Her demeanor was just all cock-eyed and un-Bev-like.

"I already did," she said very softly.

"Did what? What the hell did you do?"

"I told him I was in a relationship. Are you happy? I got sick of the harassment, feeling alone or just being alone, so I just made up a relationship."

"So what did you say? I'm sure whatever you did, it doesn't rate tears. For Christ's sake, I hope you picked a three-hundred-pound guy with martial art skills, or did you pick a cop? There's a good idea. Tell me you picked a cop. That would have been smart, or did you pick . . ." I hesitated to think of the right kind of people she should have picked, and I glanced up at her. Her expression said it all. "Oh, fuck no. Really? You did that? Tell me you didn't do that."

"Yeah, I did. Sorry," and there was another tear. I watched it slide slowly from Bev's eye to the corner of her mouth. I traced it down, and there was that thought again. I imagined it tasted a little salty and warm. She turned her head away and wiped her hand across her face.

"So now what?" I was at a loss.

"How the fuck do I know? Are you sure you don't know some kind of wheelchair karate or have a wheelchair that shoots semi-lethal bullets?" she laughed in that throaty way that made me hire her in the first place, and I couldn't help but smile.

"No such luck. I can only threaten him with getting his ass kicked out of the bar, which you had to do if I'm not mistaken." She turned back and looked at me then, and she started laughing. I followed suit. We laughed it out for another couple of minutes, then she apologized again, and I told her sincerely that there was nothing to feel sorry for, and I was flattered. I was surprised but still flattered. "Boy, you sure picked a winner," and we laughed a little more as she went about her bar routine. First, she cut up lemons and limes, then filled one of the small troughs with those god-awful maraschino cherries. Who orders those things? And then she filled up another little plastic trough with pickled onions, and I knew who ordered those, and suddenly it felt right that she had picked me. We had spent months and months together. Me, just sitting there, the penultimate fool-on-a-stool, and her, the wise bartender with a heart of gold, and an uncanny way of listening without judging. We talked about everything, from parties we had both attended that involved cocaine-filled nights and shared magic mushroom experiments. All the traveling we would do if we were rich—everything from life's ambitions to high school fumbling sexual encounters.

"Thanks," I said.

"Don't mention it. It wasn't a hard choice; slim pickings around here. I just didn't think it was going to become a pissing contest. I didn't figure the both of you being in the same room carping at each other. It's turned out to be a little weird."

"That was a given because I kind of work here too, although I know someone who might argue that point. What do you mean 'slim pickings'? For the record, it would have given me great pleasure to beat the living shit out of asshole Brian."

"Uh, right, he's like two hundred pounds plus, and he's a tough fucker. A farm boy who fights dirty."

"So was I, well not a farm boy, but I was a tough fucker in my mind, I won a 'So You Think You're Tough' contest, and that wasn't easy, let me tell you," and since she was a bartender, she knew I was going to tell her this story whether she listened or not. She poured me a very stiff martini with extra onions and the slightest trickle of sweet pickled onion juice. It's all in the details.

"Okay," she said, "I'll bite. What is a, what did you call it? A 'So You Think You're Tough' contest?"

"It was a long time ago, but back then it was a big deal. They got banned in the States for it being cruel and unusual, and they brought the whole show to Canada. They signed up all the wannabe tough guys in Vancouver and the Lower Mainland that wanted to beat the shit out of each other with tiny little gloves and not a lot of rules."

"You signed up for that shit? Sorry, it's just that you seem more of a surfer dude who would sit on a beach in California drinking Coronas with limes."

"Nope, I was a mean, skinny, tall fucker, and I enjoyed a good fight. Okay, I didn't love it per se. I was just good at it. My sister pretty much summed it up when she said I had poor impulse control. Every other weekend, whether it was defending a friend or being a bad drunk, it was fight-night, so I figured, why not give this 'So You Think You're Tough' contest a go."

"What was the big draw? I've still got you working on your tan and making football bets."

"I don't know. I wanted to prove myself and beat up bikers, bouncers, and other people who thought they were good at fighting. I've taken my share of bad beatings, usually from some fucker who kicked me in the face when I was down, usually someone not even in the fight. In the end, you could win a thousand bucks, which was not bad cash ten years ago. I guess I always liked boxing and karate. I wondered if I was decent at either."

"Yeah, my brother was a boxer. The one living with me, trying to be a nurse, go figure. He even tried to get his Golden Gloves but fell a little short. It kept him out of trouble. It sounds like this contest was more of a bunch of nut-balls just trying to beat the crap out of each other. Amateur idiots. How many rounds and how many fights?"

"Not all amateurs. You could pick out the ring-savvy dudes, guys that knew what they were getting into, and it was four fights in one night. Each fight was three rounds of three minutes, if it went that far. Every round was the longest three minutes of my life."

"So, you won this thing?" She sounded interested, so I continued. Neither one of us was going anywhere.

"Yep, four fights that never made it past the second round against guys built like brick shithouses mostly, some nice guys just trying to make a buck. It was a long night of fear, sweat, and a locker room smell that never leaves you. Everyone was cocky and full of themselves. You'd think they were a pack of pit bulls instead of scared fucks full of false bravado and bullshit. It's kinda funny when you look back on it. I really had no idea what I was getting into, but there I was in the line to sign up, and it was a parade of guys with tattoos and big rings. These were guys trying to make a name for themselves. I was a guy from Maple Ridge wearing an old ragged, loud Hawaiian shirt, with a four dollar pair of rubber thongs on my feet. I got fortunate, though, because some gym owner picked me out of the lineup, gave me a business card, and asked me if I wanted to come down to his gym and train for a month before the contest."

"Why did he pick you?"

"Don't sound so surprised, but I honestly don't know because I wasn't that special. The little man gave the same card to probably five or six other guys in the lineup. Tony Dowling, Irish gym owner, boxing promoter, pimp. His gym was right in welfare central around Main and Hastings, the skids in Vancouver, a neighborhood full of strip bars, junkies, whores, and homeless people. You had to walk over condoms and needles to get to the front door. I went because I wasn't doing much of anything else productive. I was sitting in a lawn chair at Alouette Lake, drinking a Styrofoam cooler full of beer every day with many like-minded individuals enjoying unemployment insurance."

"So, basically drinking your life away with directionless fuck-ups who were not unlike yourself."

"Hey, slow down there. It was a discovery phase. Anyway, I go to this guy's gym and see two other guys from the sign-up line. He takes us all into the office and tells us it's an investment in his time, but if one of us won the contest, we'd allow him to promote us. So I signed some silly hunk of paper that absolved him of any blame should we get injured permanently or die."

"So what, you're like two hundred pounds? You look like you might be about two hundred on a good day before the wheelchair thing."

"Fuck no, I was maybe a shade under one-ninety. I peaked at about two-ten a long time later, but I was still growing. One-eighty was lightweight. Two divisions, heavyweight and lightweight, and I wasn't stepping into a ring with an angry three-hundred-pound biker looney tune with little gloves on. I figured I could lose nine or ten pounds in a month. So I skipped rope in a sauna with friggin' garbage bags on. It's hard to lose that weight when you're six feet tall. I was going for a Michael Spinks thing, and next thing you know, you've got headgear on and you're sparring with every weight class in the gym, with this Dowling guy yelling at you every step of the way. With his Irish accent. I can still hear him, 'C'mon you feckin' gobshites, you 'it like lettle girls and ahld wahmen, you useless twats,' but I sure learned a lot of boxing shit in a hurry."

"I'm getting the drift, you ain't the light-heavy-weight title guy, but you got a little instruction, and a real boxer would have punched your clock, but you learned just enough to win," said Bev, still sounding skeptical.

"Yeah, way to shorten it, quit high jacking my glory story. So every fight was different, and the first one was with one of the guys I trained with at the gym. I felt I could beat him because he couldn't get out of his own head. He thought the whole thing was a tea party and everyone would just touch gloves and spar. I was there because I didn't mind hurting people. There were no dirty shots, no low-blows, but it wasn't like playing tag in the sparring ring, and there was no headgear. He had a dumb look on his face, and I smacked him senseless in a round and a half, and I didn't feel bad. Next up."

"You're going to give me a round for round update, aren't you?"

"I was planning on it. Mix me another martini, and I'll get into more details."

"What did you say about my bull-riding story? Oh yeah, 'Will wonders never cease,' like I was just another redneck bull-riding chick, and let me tell you, that wasn't easy either but go ahead. You realize you've had three martinis already, and we haven't even opened the doors."

"I said that? 'Will wonders never cease?' Well, I'm an asshole, and how do I know when we open? I never touch those doors. I just come in the back, where it says Staff Entrance."

"Maybe we'll talk about that later, what your responsibilities are, but yeah, go ahead, where am I going next?"

"Okay, so the next guy is a lot tougher. He hit me hard enough to see stars, but I kept dancing, more like shuffling. But the thing is, every time I hit *him*, he just held his hands up and turned around like it was a scheduled break. He did it twice, and finally I just hit him in the back of his head, not hard, just to let him know I wasn't happy with it, and the crowd booed me."

"Bet you hated that?"

"Yeah, funny but you wanted the crowd to like you. I don't know why. So this guy gets warned, and I get warned, no hitting in the back of the head. So, I hit him again with a good left jab in the beak, and he throws up a hand, holds his nose, and turns around again, and this part I'm not proud of, but I run around the front of him and smack him again. He keeps turning, and I run around, trying to get in front of him and pop him with a good one. It probably looked pretty funny. This time the crowd kind of cheers and boos. Then I quit caring and don't give him a chance to hold his hands up. I just keep punching from everywhere until he goes down, and the ref steps in and stops it when he does go down on one knee, still holding up a hand like he wants to answer a question in grade school. That whole fight took another round and a half."

"Good going, killer."

"I'm still gonna tell you this, so fuck you, Miss Judgy. I'm making it sound easier than it was. The third guy was a boxer. I mean, he stood there like one and kept jabbing away. He hit me, but you're so jacked up on adrenaline that you don't feel the little jabs, and he's got no follow-up. But halfway through round two, I caught him with a left hook, and he went down like a sack of hammers, glass jaw or something, and I feel it. I feel like I can beat anybody. The final guy . . ."

"Hang on, hero. I'm going to mix a drink."

"No, mine's still pretty full."

"Not for you jackass, for me. You are now officially paying me to listen, and we'll discuss my raise later."

"Okay, tough audience. So, the final thousand-dollar, winner-takes-all fight comes up. We both had to go to the same dressing room while they hyped the fight, and this guy was a total douche. I want to touch gloves and say good luck, but he tells me to fuck off. I mean, he's maybe five-foot-eight, but he is built like a fire hydrant, and I can tell he's already dismissed me. My family and friends in the stands are thinking the same thing; they've seen three of his elimination fights already, and they think I don't stand a chance. He keeps looking at me like I had just puked in his new car. 'Fuck you,' was his answer to everything. I reminded myself that we had to endure three fights to get to this point. I belonged in the same dressing room. I learned later he was a bouncer at the Drake, a notorious strip bar frequented by bikers and assholes and puffed-up bodybuilders of the finest kind. In short, he was more than a handful, but we had both come through to the final the same way. So I said, 'Fuck you, too,' and I tried to look tough. I know I was getting massively pissed off."

"And how did that go?" said Bev, smiling. At least she is still listening while I'm doing my Bruce Springsteen glory days bullshit.

"Well, I heard later that my good friend Danny Shea had bet a hundred against me because he had watched the human fire hydrant destroy three guys, but I hadn't watched, and to me, he was just another guy in a ring. By this time, Dowling had become my ringside trainer. He gave me more advice as I sat on my little stool, waiting for the fight to start. 'He's a stocky little gobshite,' he says, 'I'll give the fecker that. It's too bad you can't just kick him in the snookers. He's a brawler though, so keep your distance.'

"'That's your advice?' I asked him. "'Kick him in the snookers?'"

"'No, no,' he says. 'Joehst stay ooeht o' reach, and you shooehld be ahkay, maybe jab wit yooehr right instead o' yooehr left. Cahnfuse 'im. 'E doesn't look te smart.'" I took a big sip of my martini, proud of my newfound Irish accent, and I watched her make us both triple martinis before the first customer came through the door. She's drinking Gibson's martinis, too; whether she likes them or not is something I don't ask, but it's adorable. It gives me a warm feeling inside, but that could be the martinis.

"Okay," I say, martinis in hand, and we do a quick click of glasses. "Cheers," I said, and we both drank half in one sip.

"And then some," she says with a smile that shows all the laugh lines around her eyes.

"So, to continue," I say, the warm feeling of gin before noon in my stomach, winding up for the big finish. "I didn't fully understand a single fucking thing Dowling said, except to stay out of reach. How the hell can you win at boxing by staying out of reach? So instead, I waded in, and strangely enough, there was that feeling. I took three deep breaths and thought about baseball, hockey, and swimming. Then I thought, the guy in front of you was just another opponent, and you're here for a reason. You want that thousand bucks more than he does, and he wouldn't even touch gloves before the fight. He pissed me right off. It was just another fight. Oh, he tagged me. He hit me with a kidney shot that had me ultimately in bed pissing blood for a week. Then I got a shot to the chin where I figured I would've lost a half-dozen teeth if not for the mouthguard I was wearing. It was a battle, but Dowling was no dummy, and a month in the gym came back to me. I got cocky, only a little, but you need a little cocky when it's you in the ring, you and one other guy. A guy who bled just like you. So I jabbed twice like I had done one thousand times in the gym, only this time with my right and then an uppercut with the left. Dowling had called that move. 'Get in-between 'is elbows,' he said, 'go southpaw and do sahme chin knahckin.' So in desperation or otherwise, I followed his advice. I staggered the fire hydrant, and fuck me, like I was going to let him get a second wind. I descended on him like a crazed buzzsaw. I went all Aaron Pryor on his ass and didn't quit until the ref pulled me off. In the end, the thousand dollars was mine, and he was crumpled. He was on one knee against the ropes in the corner. After the referee stopped it, I tried to help him up, but he wanted none of that. He looked at me with unabashed hatred. He made me want to hit him again. That aside, it was the coolest thing I ever did. I won a thousand bucks, and the fights and stories came. It was broadcast all across Canada. My parents were on Texada Island in B.C. watching Tony Parsons and the evening news with some friends, and there was their son with his hands in the air jumping around like a lunatic cause he beat a bunch of people up. Even my future in-laws in Ontario saw the show. So it was pretty cool, my fifteen minutes of fame. Kinda fucked up, though. I had to fight many people after that because they thought it was a fluke. My buddy, Mike Bignell, was supposed to tape it, but he fucked up the time thingy, a.m., p.m., whatever, so you'll just have to take my word for it."

"So, as you would say, 'there's a moral in every story.' What's the moral in this one, Mr. Aesop?"

"I don't know. No morals, I guess . . . I wish I could still beat up assholes, and it frustrates me beyond reason that I can't. Maybe 'accept your fate,' which is a moral I just made up, and Aesop I ain't."

"Hey, life goes on. It is what it is."

"That is your entire bartender wisdom about my story and my condition, 'Life goes on,' and, 'It is what it is'?"

"Yeah, we're all just little people trying to get by. I'm glad you got your fifteen minutes of fame. I'm still looking for mine. It's a great story, but it doesn't mean that's all you are. You're better than one story. It is maybe a defining moment in your old life, but it's not why I put up with you," and she downed the rest of her martini in one swallow. Finally, the doors were open, and people drifted in. I half-filled my wineskin and went home to watch football, and maybe bet on a game or two.

CHAPTER FORTY-ONE

MORE DEPRESSION, HIDDEN DEPRESSION

TWO DAYS LATER, I TALKED to my money partners—a couple of brothers, the Georges—from Peace River and Grande Prairie (they owned Boston Pizzas at these locations). Good people who were just watching the bottom line. They worried about the amount of spillage at the bar and all the advertising we were doing to get our restaurant off the launching pad. They were reasonable men, but they were a little pissed off about the money going out instead of the money coming in. I was only getting paid a thousand bucks a month, and I was feeling pissy, so 'fuck them and their spillage problem' was my attitude.

It was another slow afternoon, a Tuesday, and I was already three sheets to the wind. I was into my sixth martini, drinking a beer out of one of the few carnival mugs still left over from the promo. Bev had joined me earlier than usual, same big ass mug, same cold Canadian. Usually she would sip on a Long Island iced tea or a margarita—she'd given up martinis—but today she was pounding them down pretty good. She was very introspective, not talking much, just flipping the bill of my hat and smiling. We were doing a lot of "glass clinking."

"What's eating you?" I asked, because bartenders also needed someone to talk to and I had become an avid listener, but I was on the edge of being drunk and entirely past the point where I could advise if necessary.

"It's that fuckhead Brian. It's turning into more than a stalking thing."

"I got nothing, kid, never been there. Generally, after every relationship I've ever had, the other party hates my guts, just saying," and while I was just saying, who should walk into the bar on some kind of fucked up cue but asshole Brian. He was glassy-eyed, crazed-looking, and drunk but too aware. No stumbles, no hesitation, just looking shiny and sweating buckets. I had been there, done that and could spot it a mile away. He was coked up to the eyeballs and was more like a walking zombie, but this time he sat on a stool barely five feet away from my space.

"Gimp," he said by way of greeting. Big shit-eating grin and a nod in my direction, the barest evidence of white powder on the end of one nostril. One big snort in the parking lot before coming in half-cocked.

"Fuckhead," I countered. Mike Bignell in my head once again, saying, "Nothing good could come of this." He sucked at taping shit, but he did have some good sayings, much like the rest of the pack I hung around with most of my life.

"Fuck you, gimp," he says louder with a big sneer. "So, you got a thing for Bev, I hear. What's the problem, no gimp chicks around?"

"Okay, that's enough," chirped up Bev, trying to defuse the situation. Mike Bignell and his little saying must have been in her head too. I was a little pissed that she felt the need to defend me, making me feel reckless.

"Yeah, I got a thing for Bev, fuckhead. What are you gonna do about it?" I asked, getting all puffy. This situation was spinning out of control in a big hurry.

"Hey, I'd punch the shit out of you, gimp, and I wouldn't feel guilty for a second. But easy for you, being a brave little man behind the bar, you gonna get Bev to call the cops again?" Bev had apparently called the cops on him more than once, whether it was for stalking or just being a drunk prick. At the time it didn't matter.

I pondered the question for about eight seconds, and then that poor impulse control thing popped up. "Have at 'er then, fuckhead," I said, like that was some weird battle cry. I turned Bert to high and he was three hundred pounds of furious metal, batteries, and motors and with me attached. I came out from the corner of the bar—four miles an hour—like my wheelchair was possessed. I ran right over him and his silly stool and the one behind it, and he landed four feet away on his ass. I was trying like hell to get unstuck from the stool and the foot rail so I could take another run. My chair had jumped up when I smacked into his stool. The son of a bitch made it to his feet faster than I thought he would, and he was on me, swinging wildly. I dodged the first haymaker by pulling my head back, and I ducked under the next one, but my balance was all skewed from my martini and beer lunch, and I fell over my knees, and then I did the only thing I could do. I stuck my head between my knees while he pounded on my back. He stopped that at one point and was now trying to pull me out of the chair. He almost had my shirt over my head and was yanking on it like a crazed hockey player. Unfortunately for him, it was a wasted tactic. I was belted into Bert, and no amount of tugging would unseat me. He was pulling against three hundred pounds of wheelchair and about one hundred seventy pounds of Quad. It was probably the weirdest coked-up, drunken parody of a hockey fight you would ever see.

The bugger of it was there was a lot of flailing from me, without the use of my triceps and my inability to make a proper fist. So I switched tactics. I leaned on my joystick, trying to go forward. I could hear the wheels spinning and the smell of burned rubber on the tiles, but I was bound and determined to run him over again, so now I'm rocking back and forth like I'm riding a mechanical bull, trying hard to get the wheelchair unstuck, and my head is down between my knees again. Finally, I hear a big *THUNK* like the dull side of an ax hitting a chopping block. Time stands still, and then the weight of his body falls on my back. I quit struggling after that, and I'm trying to push my body upright, but Brian is goddamned heavy. Bev was right when she said he's a bit of a solid load. Then another *THUNK*, and Brian slowly slides off. He is now lying at my feet, close to unconsciousness. Blood is spilling down his face in little streams, and he's mumbling unintelligibly. He's babbling insensate and trying to crawl to his feet, but the best he can do is hold onto my pantlegs and my shoes while he bleeds all over the floor.

My head comes up then, and I twist in my chair to look behind me. There is Bev. She's got an insane look on her face, and it is not the look of a woman in control of her emotions.

She's got her arm up, and I can see the Giant Mug at about one o'clock. As much as I want her to smoke Brian one more time, I could see that it was totally unnecessary. He had a colossal scalp laceration and was now lying on my feet, bleeding and mumbling. "Whoa, whoa, stop. He's done. Slow down and put down the mug," I say before she kills him.

"Fuck you. Just one more hit and I don't have to deal with this cock-sucker ever again," she says between clenched teeth.

"He ain't worth it, man. Look at him. I think you might have fucking killed him already. Phone an ambulance. This guy is bleeding all over my Stan Smiths. He is not a threat anymore. I don't know? Maybe wash the Giant Mug in your hand. It's got, like, blood and hair stuck to it. But, holy shit, how hard did you hit this guy?"

"As hard as I could. I was saving your ass and trying to kill his, a two-for-one deal."

"One shot would have saved my ass, that second shot was all you, and the third shot would have been the jailhouse shot, as in you'd be going to jail for murder. Please wash the Giant Mug." I'm strangely calm now. That always happens after the big head rush of adrenaline.

"No way. I'm putting it on the fucking wall, right next to your hubcap." She had calmed herself down, but her hands were visibly shaking. She sucked down the fourteen ounces of beer still left in my wonderfully thought-out Giant Mug. The usual inscrutable Bev look was on her face again, and she was already dialing the phone. Brian had stopped mumbling by this time, and he was just lying there bleeding a lot. Blood was pooling by my feet as we silently waited for an ambulance. Words didn't seem to matter and thank Christ that it is not a busy day. Tammy the waitress hadn't arrived yet, and my wife was busy doing the end of the lunch rush, herding cats dressed up as waitresses. "Maybe we should hide the body," Bev says.

"What are you, some kind of fucking serial killer now? What's next? Cut him into pieces? I got a better idea. Get yourself a strong drink, pour me another martini, and let's hope like hell that he doesn't bleed to death.

Maybe you should like, I don't know, hold a towel on his head, check his pulse, I don't know, what the fuck."

"I'm not touching him. Just leave him there. If he starts talking, I'll hit him again," and it does occur to me that there is nothing I can do. So we both get Bert unstuck by rocking back and forth, scarring the brass rail with scratches and dents, forever mementos to a strange barroom fight. I slowly go back to my spot behind the bar. Bev makes a couple of drinks, and luckily restaurant drink orders aren't coming in, so we both stare at each other and drink like Brian isn't even there. It's freaky. It almost feels like we should be talking about the weather, the stock market, or silly things while calmly enjoying an afternoon cocktail. It doesn't take long for the ambulance to come. It's the direct opposite of what you want to see when opening a new restaurant; a big white van with flashing lights. Man, that was fast. I'm guessing there's not much happening in Airdrie on a Tuesday afternoon. So much for cutting him into pieces. Now we're going to have to get our heads together and explain this one away, or maybe tell the truth; that Brian is a total asshole, and he deserved to have his head smashed in with a five-pound promo twenty-four-ounce Giant Beer Mug.

Of course, my wife comes in, and why wouldn't she? "What the hell happened here?" she says, looking at bleeding Brian lying in front of the bar as Bev and I get a tequila shot. She has decided this will go well with tequilas. The stretcher comes through the restaurant opening, the wrong door, and they have to turn right around to get into the bar portion. Discreet, they are not; the stretcher is banging off the side of the entrance to the bar, and finally, my wife goes down the two stairs to the bottom portion and holds the door. Bev has kept the bottle of tequila in her hand the whole time as she pours us another shooter, and we stand there like department store mannequins, unfazed by the guy bleeding all over the floor on the other side of the bar.

The good news is that Brian has a pulse. He's picked up with a backboard and strapped into the stretcher, and they whisk him away with very little fanfare. Very little fanfare if you're used to ambulances appearing during a quiet lunch with the siren on and the lights on. They asked his name and the circumstances, and they never looked behind the bar. The Giant Mug is sitting there on the lower shelf with dried blood and a couple of hairs still sticking to it. My wife has taken over. Bev and I sit there like wooden statues watching a bad movie playing out. They are gone in what seems like minutes, with no cops. They've stopped the fanfare. Sirens off, lights still spinning, silently, like it's all done, everybody gets on with their day, nothing to see here. My wife has explained that he slipped out of his stool because he was drunk and smacked his head on the tile floor. Just bad luck, she says, even though it doesn't explain how he's got *two* big gashes on his head. After all, he didn't bash his head on the floor once and then do it again because it felt so good the first time. My wife is somewhat aware of who Brian is, and she stares at us like a couple of unruly teenagers. Bev starts taking her apron off.

"What do you think you're doing?" says my wife in a stern, no-nonsense voice. The one she uses when she's training particularly stubborn waitresses.

"Cashing out, I figured you'd be firing me," says Bev with a big sigh, sounding defeated.

"Fuck that," I finally pipe up like an idiot fan behind the glass at a hockey game where you feel safe poking the bear. "She should get a raise." This comment rewards me with a look that could cut diamonds, and I shut my mouth and become a spectator again, but I'm not backing down on this one. My wife senses this. She comes around from behind the bar, and her tone softens.

"Bev, I'm sure you had a reason, so we will get our story straight. That idiot sitting beside you should take right off after you spray his runners off near the drain and wash that fucking special beer mug." After that calm speech, she looks at me directly and tells me to fuck off, but not in so many words. It is really not hard to gauge her opinion of me at this point. I don't want this turning into a management face-off in front of the restaurant patrons and the gathered staff. They stand there like fucking seagulls at a garbage dump, waiting for their next meal. I quietly ask Bev to fill my wineskin from the keg of house wine on tap. She does this without comment and puts it over my head, and the pregnant leather skin feels weighty on my chest, heavy and full of promise to someone who just wants to get the hell out of there and put Bert on cruise control. Bev also squeezes my thigh real hard, I don't care who sees this, and she says, "Don't worry, I got your back," and I think that should be my line, but off I go through the swinging doors at the servants' entrance and out of the restaurant to quietly ponder my future.

CHAPTER FORTY-TWO

STEP FOUR AND A HALF

SO HERE I AM, THREE-HUNDRED and thirty-six days since I crashed the trusty Mojave Toyota truck into a drainage ditch. I am as drunk as a newt, and I hate myself. I still hated "rude." I wanted to be that cocky swinging, no quit, no excuses, hard-man. But this was not the case. No, this was clearly not the case, and I was supposed to swallow my ego and realize my circumstances: me and my trusty wineskin.

Bev has my back. It hit me like a sucker punch in the gut, and the blood drained from my face. I felt shame. I felt helpless. Welcome to your new life, gimpy Quad-boy. Your fate is to be a footnote in the fall from grace category. My cross to bear, no more three-round contests, no fights, no defense, no stance save phone the cops, and turtle, just turtle. Another unbidden memory had surfaced as I shut up and stewed blue, sitting in my wheelchair in my little spot by the bar as Bev filled my sneaky wineskin. Just another fucked up memory while I stood in the corner like a recalcitrant child, and I felt pounded. I think this flashback was the one that tipped the scales. This helped me get to step four and a half.

I played hockey when I was fifteen and was initially picked for the Rep Team. It was the same players year in and year out. There were no "going to the show" players, just guys who were better than average and learned how to skate faster or shoot straighter. I knew every one of those guys: the Milos, the Baileys, the Townsends, the Shellborns, and the Walkers, the list goes on. They kicked me off that team because of my bad attitude, the fighting, and being a goofball. So I was busted back to the House League, scoring goals by the pantload, and it was a fun team. No one took themselves too seriously, and there were no Westwoods and Meyers and Kirkwoods thinking they would be called up to the bigs any day now.

So every time the other team got behind, they would target me. Taking out one of the best guys is a tried-and-true Canadian hockey strategy. Their bruiser goon would goad me into a fight, and it didn't take much prompting as I was highly goadable. That, and that damned impulse control thingy.

I had lost track of how many hockey fights I had long ago, but I never learned, so I would spend five minutes thinking about it in the penalty box way too often. But one day, the coach pulled me aside and told me, "Just turtle. Tuck your legs in, cover your head, and wait for the refs to break it up. You're one of our best players and they're trying to get you in the box, so don't be an idiot and lose your ego. Be a team player. Take one for the team."

I did it just once. It was humiliating, turtling, laying on the ice with my legs tucked in and my head covered with my gloves, feeling nothing but anger and shame while some goon smacked me around like a pinata. It all flooded back, an unbidden memory about turtling because I couldn't help but be a turtle now. The rest of my life stretched out ahead of me, and I realized that a turtle was all I was ever going to be. You betcha, a real-life fucking, honest-to-goodness turtle, just tuck your little legs in and cover your head. So, off I went that fateful afternoon, holding back tears. Frustration is a powerful emotion. I guess the cops were coming to the restaurant, and I was told more or less to "fuck off," for a good reason; being the undisputed king of day drinking, I did that very thing. I was already drunk, and my afternoon was already planned. I hugged my good friend, the wineskin, and went on another walkabout.

I drove, just me and Bert, my dependable companion, who knew me better than anybody. Okay, yes, I personified the fucking chair. I spent every hour of every day counting on my friend Bert, and that day was no exception. I went down roads, paved trails, and paths. I took advantage of the golf course close to the restaurant, the same golf course where they had offered me a discount membership in another life, and I slowly cruised all eighteen holes, just motoring down the pathway with little regard for golfing etiquette. Neither did I give a flying fuck about golf balls or the people yelling at me. I should still have had the hubcap duct-taped to my head, but that was back at the restaurant, presumably hanging on the wall with Bev's Giant Mug.

I was deep in thought. I would stop periodically, watch a foursome hit on a par three, and have another drink from the wineskin. It held thirty ounces of deliciously sour white wine, and it took me ten miles to drink it dry. Every mile brought me closer to the inevitable. The curse of the inevitable had me in its grasp. I was never going to be the man I once was. I was never going to be in control of my life. Instead, my life now controlled me.

I eventually headed for my tiny apartment. I had things to do because, during my walkabout, I had made up my mind. There was no one home, of course. My wife was due back when she finished at the restaurant, whenever that was, I wasn't looking forward to seeing her. It was around four in the afternoon, so I had seven, eight, or more hours of feeling sorry for myself. She stayed at the restaurant later and later, the usual excuse, playing darts and hanging with the staff. Something I couldn't do, and it hit home that my wife and I were already estranged, already just going through the motions. The game was long over, but we couldn't quite get to the finish. It was like playing solitaire, and you're out of options, but what the hell, let's flip over the deck one more time to see if something magically changed.

I ran out of wine at about the same time I arrived home. I went up the wheelchair ramp, punched in the door code, and navigated the entrance-way. Once inside, I pulled out a mug and filled it with warm vodka. Then, I searched for and found my little portable cassette, the miniature hand-held version, and I inserted a new tape, fresh out of the sealed package. It even smelled new. I loved the smell of new stuff, a new book, or the rubbery smell of a new pair of Stan Smiths. Yesiree, new smells for an old, old life.

My head was reeling. I felt completely and utterly drunk, and I had so much to say and wisdom to impart to those closest to me, only it wouldn't come. I didn't feel wise or prophetic. I didn't feel anything. I rolled over to the large window in the living room where the sun came in the late after-noon. It was warm and bright, a beautiful spring day, and I could see the Rocky Mountains in the distance. I wondered how many times I had been over those mountains. How many times I had grabbed a pack of "travel-ers" and drove the twelve hours to my tiny hometown of Maple Ridge, back when traveling opened up your whole life to new experiences and new memories. When you packed a small gym bag and a full cooler, you were good to go—before the accident. Now I had a three-hundred-pound wheelchair, a commode chair, a raft of medical equipment, and a broken body that had to be hand-loaded. No drop and go, no fly by the seat of your pants.

I took another large pull of warm vodka in the end, it burned going down, but it got me over the hump and bolstered my determination. I turned my tape recorder on and started my eulogy. I talked to my wife, apologizing for messing up her whole life, crashing the truck, and blowing up our future plans, for being a drunk and not having the strength of char-acter to keep on rolling any longer. I talked to my close friends, who I grew up with and loved like brothers. I spoke to my family, making excuses for what might be conceived as my cowardice. After a slow start, the words flew like they had wings. It was like I was a man deprived of an audience for years, telling a long story with no beginning or end. I talked until the tape ran out, thirty minutes of life with no regrets, memories that stretched for miles, places, and people that made up a life well-lived. Friends, too many to count, enough to fill a church, I hoped, standing room only, a litany of memories and smiles and shenanigans. Finally, I turned the tape over, refilled my mug, and rambled on again about nothing. Ragged memories, some ripped from my soul, some bittersweet, and some that made me smile and laugh aloud. I finally ran out of gas, no more rounds to fight, no more things to prove. A wilted balloon with a slow leak. It was time to shut up. Either get on with the business of living or get on with the business of dying.

I could transfer my ass into bed at this point, so I had a plan. It was a simple plan, take as many drugs as possible and go to bed for the last sleep. It was not a Cinderella poison apple plan, and nobody was going to come along and kiss me back to life, which always sounded kind of creepy anyway in a necrophilia way. Nope, my plan had no mulligans, and it was foolproof. I had enough drugs to kill an elephant, settling on this as my last act. Shooting myself was a non-starter. I had no gun. I suppose I could have used Bert to drive my sorry ass down to the railway tracks to get hit by a train, as they passed by every hour only a half block from the apartment, but Bert didn't deserve that fate—I told you I personified him.

I refilled my pint glass of vodka one last time, Grey Goose, nothing but the best for me. There was no saving it for another occasion as I didn't plan on having one. I chased down one hundred fifty milligrams of Valium, a handful of Baclofen—they were anti-spasm drugs, but I supposed they had overdose potential because they were prescription drugs. I took eight hundred milligrams of Elavil; I knew these had great overdose potential, so I swallowed all I had. I capped it off with six or seven Advil, and then I ran out of both drugs and Grey Goose. I left the little tape deck right in the middle of the kitchen table, put my favorite mixed tape in the stereo, which specifically had no Gypsy Kings on it, and emptied my piss bag. I don't know why I would empty my piss bag. I guess I wanted to preserve my dignity, and it just wouldn't do to piss myself.

I finally transferred my sorry ass to bed; my head was surprisingly clear for a guy that had consumed a bathtub full of booze and every drug in the house. I had no regret or remorse. I laid my head on the pillow and waited for my version of the last sleep. I knew it would come unbidden. It certainly did when I crashed my truck and became a burden to the rest of the world. I had time to reflect; drugs and booze don't kill you like a bullet, they take time, but I could feel my body getting lighter. I was floating again. Looking down on myself much like I did when I first got into this mess. I felt free from all the future indignities I might face, free from all the turtling I might have to do. Not once did I think of where this was going. I thought of it as an end, not the beginning of a new life without pain and strife. Nothing mystical or magical would occur, and I started counting my breaths, wondering which one might be the last.

CHAPTER FORTY-THREE

STEP ONE, AGAIN: DENIAL, FULL CIRCLE BACK TO DENIAL, BUT A HEALTHY DENIAL

IT IS PAINFULLY APPARENT THAT my plans went awry. It wasn't because I didn't take enough drugs or skimp on the alcohol. Instead, it was chance, fate, an un-fortuitous coincidence, karma, and all of those silly things we ascribe to if God is off the table, and he's never sat at mine. So I'm going to go with bad timing.

Marie, again, was the home support worker who could never leave well enough alone. She was out walking her dog that evening and just decided to drop in for a visit. Marie was like that, take a chance I might be home, drop by for a chat, make some coffee or tea, and watch her dog fight with my wife's cat, the cat with no tail; the mystery remains where the cat lost it. As I said, Marie was a beautiful person inside and out, a genuinely good person, so thinking back, I regret she had to deal with what she saw. I was well into my overdose protocol. There was a foam coming out of my mouth, and I had turned a sickly pale color, was sweating buckets, and my eyes had rolled back into my skull. I will always feel bad that she, of all people, had to deal with that mess.

As it was related to me, the ambulance came in record time (they were three streets away, having a coffee at a cafe), probably the same guys that dropped Brian off after he got cold-cocked by a Giant Mug. Luckily, or unluckily, they had plenty of Narcan or charcoal or whatever they gave to overdose monkeys. They shot me up, charged up their portable paddles at one point because of my sketchy heart rhythm (I am now aware I have a heart murmur, but apparently that's not uncommon), and they made me puke, and boy, was I made to puke. I went from dead to alive in record time, awake and shouting like I required an exorcism. They wheeled me into the hospital in Calgary, and not without incident. They tied me down to the stretcher, where I pulled on my restraints, yelled obscenities, and threatened to kill everyone. Veins bulging, head-spinning, and pissed off to be alive. Once there, they pumped my stomach and filled me with more charcoal, and, ironically, they eventually shot me up with Ativan (valium) to calm me down.

I passed out and woke up or became aware of my surroundings, bleary, sore, tired, and spent, an empty vessel, as if I had just run for days and days and hit the wall. All the muscles in my body (the ones I could still control) were on fire. I had struggled mightily and violently with my restraints, as mightily as a Quad can struggle, but I felt it.

There were bruises and fingerprint marks on my arms where they tried to hold me down. My handcuffs, or tie-downs, cut into my wrists like little knives abrading my skin where the blood had congealed around them. It felt like I had bicep curled a couple of hundred pounds ten times, until my biceps were screaming and all the tendons had snapped. My head was full of hate, and I wanted to hurt anyone within ten feet of me. I pounded on the bed like a man still possessed, yelling at nothing and no one. I was just screaming and thrashing.

It reached a point where I could barely lift my head, and every try left my neck tingling with a teeth-grinding electric shock—it was like being tasered—and the lights hurt my eyes. Everything hurt my eyes, they were dry and felt like they were each rubbed with a handful of sand, but it all returned to me. I wasn't supposed to be here, I was supposed to be dead, and as much as this felt close to death, it wasn't the death I was looking for when I started this ball rolling.

My eyes gradually focused as the hours passed, and my muddled sensibilities slowly followed suit. I was looking at fluorescent lights again, rows filled with the same fucking dead flies and distressing memories. I was back, back in the place I vowed never to return. Calgary General Hospital, where I could smell the disinfectant, the bleach, and the hopelessness. I was back full circle to where my old life had ended.

I tested my restraints once more, tried to lift my head again, and realized this was futile and beyond frustrating. They had stopped me, and someone had intervened. Someone had fucked up my master plan. I would kill them; I would hate them forever. I had been reduced to a pitiful creature that had tried and failed to commit suicide. A sideshow freak, a flop, my ultimate demise was now just a gesture, a call for help. I fucking hated life, and I imagined I would hate the coming hours even more because people would come to my room, and they would have tears in their eyes. I would be an anomaly, a fragile piece of crystal, a broken person in need of a rebuild. Everyone would be on their best behavior. I could already hear their thoughts in my damaged brain. "Don't upset the Quad. He could take something the wrong way and try to kill himself again."

And I waited and waited some more, but nobody came. No friends, no wife, no nurse, no fifty-buck-an-hour shrink (that would come later), and I was left alone with my grim thoughts. What would I do next? Strangely enough, a thousand views and new ideas came to me, suicide not being one of them. Another suicide attempt was not even a passing thought. You fail at suicide once, and there is no coming back, no do-overs. Attempting suicide was some pretty serious shit. I spent hours lying there, rethinking my life. In the end, I knew what was coming next only too well. I would be consoled, questioned, treated like a defective cog in the machine, a cracked egg that all the king's horses and all the king's men couldn't put back together again. Fuck fuckity fuck, this was not in my plans. Okay, so let's make some new plans, and it became that simple. Clarity came unbidden, but I knew my future. It was set in stone.

I had woken up and was a different person. All the bruises, the restraints, and the repercussions meant nothing to me anymore. I knew what I was going to do. I knew with such conviction that no amount of advice or consolation would stop me. I was going home; it was that simple. Disregard the last twenty-four hours. Forget about the previous ten or eleven months. It was crystal clear, my own little epiphany without the God part. Can you have an epiphany without God? I wasn't sure, but I knew the next step. It was the life raft that comes by when you're floundering in an endless ocean. I had failed miserably at killing myself, let's call it what it was, attempted suicide by drugs and booze, a failsafe combination that had somehow led to failure.

The decision on what to do next came easy. Maybe it was always there staring me right in the face. Go back to a place where you're surrounded by people who love you, people who asked nothing of you, a place where there was nothing left to prove. I had friends, family, familiarity, and all the things I needed to heal myself because it was self-evident that I was broken. I had run out of gas, a spent unit, like a burned-out bulb, and another twenty lines of mixed metaphors. Bottom line, I hated the fucking restaurant. I would never go back there. That part of my life was over.

My wife finally appeared at my bedside. She looked awful, her eyes were puffy and red, and it looked like she hadn't slept for two days. This was all to familiar. The first thing out of my mouth was, "It wasn't your fault. None of this is your fault."

"Well, how do you think I feel?" was the first thing out of her mouth.

"You probably feel guilty is my best guess," and that's the thing, the bugger of it all . . . you try to kill yourself, and everyone wants to know the why and wherefore after you try and fail to check out, and it's the most complex question to answer. It's hard to explain your detached feeling as you gulp back pills with warm vodka. It's a self-seeking attempt at calling your shitty, minor, inconsequential life quits. It's very personal and hard to convey to anyone who isn't on the same page. It was easy for me because I already knew the outcome of my new and improved life.

Trying to explain, I said, "If it helps, I feel a little guilty, but the reasoning seemed so clear when I was stuffing myself with various narcotics and washing it all down with throat-burning liquor. Now my reasons seem petty, fucking stupid, and without merit, but I know what I have to do."

"And what's that?" She sounds peevish, like she should be consulted about my new revelation. I felt judged, but why the fuck not? That selfish thing kept popping up in my brain like a tape on a loop. Was my attempt at leaving this miserable life behind selfish? Find me another poor, feeling-sorry-for-himself fuckup in a wheelchair with a primarily dead body and too many responsibilities, and I'll talk to him. I could ask him how he feels about pissing in a bag, about not being able to get an erection, unless it was a useless one that could occur at any time like a mocking little mascot. I could ask him how it felt to shit the bed while you're sleeping. It's just how it feels to watch an athletic contest where you are a forever spectator, a sideline dreamer about the "good old days." To feel so useless and pathetic when a rude, big asshole comes into a bar and you can't beat the living shit out of him or at least try. How you cry inside and outside about the person you used to be. The person you now have to kill, the person you have to erase in your mind, destroy and eliminate. The Randy Wagner you knew is now dead. He's ashes, he doesn't even cast a shadow, and now I have to rebuild myself, one step at a time. I have to put this goddamn jigsaw puzzle back together, and at least I know how to start doing that. I blurt out my intentions without thinking. It still seems so clear to me.

"I'm heading back to where I feel like I matter. I don't want to be reminded of what I can't do every day, like when I go into that fucking Boston Pizza and I don't feel like I'm contributing anything. I feel like I roll around in my chair like a disconnected specter who needs a booze jumpstart to care about being there. I was a lost soul looking for my past days as a Boston Pizza manager, where I could just jump in, make a batch of dough, save the day when the kitchen got swamped with orders, and the whole place was in the weeds. I could insert myself into that situation and make a dent, a difference." Where did that rant come from? I am rolling down a precarious highway now, but I couldn't stop; this idea has no brakes and no runoff lane. Come what may.

"I used to have a purpose," I continued, even surer of myself. "It felt good at the end of the day, like I had accomplished something. I had pride . . . now I feel like I'm in the way, like a traffic cone on a crowded highway. Fuck me. All I do is drink and make the odd decision, like if we should have the cream of broccoli soup or clam chowder. Shortly after that, I manage my drink choices between noon and seven. I either choose a martini or a pint, and I nurse my broken ego until I can go home without getting lost or flipping Bert. I get put to bed, watch a little T.V., pass out, and imagine I'm not in a wheelchair." I must admit that was a big bundle of unwrapped shit, and I wasn't sure how my wife would take it.

"Well, what do you want me to do?" she said quietly. She was crying now, and I realized my voice had risen, and I was indeed having quite a rant. It was not directed at my wife, but I am sure she felt it was.

"I'm sorry, I really am. But, as I said, it's not your fault. None of it is. It wasn't you who fell asleep and crashed the truck into a ditch. That was all me."

She looked up at me with tears and caught her voice. "So maybe you should get some help? Counseling or something."

"I just tried to kill myself to avoid that very thing. I'm just not the counseling type."

"So your intention is to leave it all behind and give it all up?"

"Yep, back to Maple Ridge. It's all yours. It was your dream in the first place, and I was just a passenger. I hopped on the restaurant train to have an ambition, even if it was someone else's dream. I wanted all this stuff to work out so you could achieve your goal in life, and don't look at me like I'm nuts. It became my dream too, in the end, my obsession, but once I got there after we scored our very own restaurant and we became owners, and I ended up in a chair, there was nothing left to do. Mission accomplished. There has to be a next."

"So what's your *next* big plan, go back to Maple Ridge? What's there? What makes that place better than this place?" I could tell she was getting a little pissed off at me, and I felt like I wasn't making my point.

"Yes, that place is better than this place. There are no expectations. It's like I need a new objective. A clean slate where I can start over."

"If that's what you want to do," and she shrugged, wiping the tears from her face. I like to think she struggled with the idea at first, but I could see the change in her demeanor, like a shade being drawn down slowly that was blocking out the light. Like the deal was done, and it was weird. She turned into Wes's fiancée.

I expected a different reaction. I hoped my wife would grab my leg and say, "Don't go." It wouldn't have mattered, but I still wanted an impassioned plea, like in the old movies where the hero is leaving, and the whole town can't do without him, and the heroine (my wife) tearfully cries my name, hoping that I might change my mind at the last minute. A "Shane" moment with tears and recriminations. This was not like that, not at all. This was a wave and a farewell, like watching an old horse and rickety wagon roll out of town with all my earthly belongings tied in the back. A rocking chair, the butter churn, the old four-poster bed, and an old dog that can't entirely run behind the wagon anymore. A sad adios, farewell, and goodbye. I hope you find a better life. Happy fucking trails.

I should have expected this. Over the last year, I had forfeited my role as a broken hero, and I had nobody left to save. I was a loser a long time ago. I just didn't know it. So our relationship gradually changed, morphing, not something you could put your finger on, just a subtle shift in the wind. But ah, fuck it, there were sails up with nothing left to fill them. They were luffing heavily. The good ship Randy Wagner was dead in the water and charting a new course.

"When do you want to leave?" she asked, letting me know she was not going to try to stop me. She knew, and I knew, this was inevitable; we had just never put it into words. Then it occurred to me that she had heard *the tape*. The fucking tape, where I had spilled my whole life out, without reservation, because I wasn't coming back. The cassette tape of crushed dreams and sorrow. Me trying to sum up my pathetic lost-cause life. I'm thinking somewhere in that messy drunken final good night, I had mentioned (more than once) that we had grown apart, and my feelings for her had taken a sharp left and kind of fallen off a cliff like little emotional lemmings, jumping to their death one behind the other. I had called her selfish, which in retrospect was dumber than dogshit. I was selfish because she had been trying to hold her life together in an environment that had changed drastically.

It was just as hard, or more complex, on her as it was on me. It was clear to me now that her one foot had been out the door long ago because life must go on. I wondered if she had already started another relationship, something to fill the void. I had dug a giant hole all by myself and neglected to make room for her. Couples (I learned later) don't usually make it through the "rebirth." You are different and they aren't. They still walk, function, and want to embrace life while you're trying to get through it one day at a time. I've lost something that can never be found again. Our sex life was good before, and now it was simply non-existent. We had not even tried to work around the wheelchair, the condom catheter, and later the indwelling one. My spontaneous hard-ons were unscheduled. A good flick of a finger right on the head of my dick could pretty much kill one, no matter how promising it looked.

I couldn't do it anymore, but let's call it what it was. It certainly wasn't my wife. It was me. I had been the strong one that you could lean on and depend on, and now I was not. It wasn't that simple, yet it was. We played the same game for nine years, a bumpy relationship that smoothed out and inevitably led to marriage, and it was just rounding into form when suddenly, I'm a wheelchair guy. It was much like the old tablecloth trick; jerk it hard enough, the plates and cutlery barely move, and you're left with a crumpled-up tablecloth. Now try to put it back. Not so easy, is it? I couldn't do it. So the last option is to clear the fucking table and start again.

I wasn't giving her what she needed because I was too caught up in my imagined insecure frailties. I had tuned out the world a long time ago. Finally, with great conviction, I realized it was time to go home again. The same friend who said that "Cold was fucking cold, humid or dry," also said, "All roads lead to Maple Ridge." I'm sure this wasn't on Larry Siemens's mind ten years ago when he said it, but it was comically apparent that he was right, right as rain in this instance. Way to go, Lar, for your insight, but it was a done deal. My road now led to Maple Ridge. Although, just as I was about to say that, the psychiatrist made his appearance.

CHAPTER FORTY-FOUR

STEP FIVE: ACCEPTANCE, REAL ACCEPTANCE

I NEVER MUCH LIKED PSYCHIATRISTS. I always thought of them as bottom feeders, people sucking up all the detritus of other people's lives and getting some kind of weird nourishment out of failure (much like Wes). Egg-crackers and head-squeezers are educated people who know nothing about suffering or real life. No matter how many books you read, you cannot beat life experience. I realize now that I planned on being combative and argumentative before the session started. At that moment, having someone pry into my life to expose my inner demons and lost dreams was beyond a waste of both my time and theirs.

He did make quite an entrance. First, all the light went out of the doorway. It was eclipsed. Then I heard a *plunk, plunk* sound like someone was using a sizeable two-headed cane. *Step, plunk, plunk, step, plunk, plunk.* He paused briefly, like walking three steps had worn him out. He came closer and the light from the hall now silhouetted a large body, slightly slumped, holding a fold-up chair in his right hand. The chair was small, and he was immense. He double plunk-stepped to my bedside without a word, unfolded, and sat down in a chair that looked better suited to a child's tea party. He heaved a big sigh, opened a tiny briefcase, shuffled a few papers, and jumped right into the deep end. "So," he said, "what's your story?" He pushed his tiny John Lennon specs up, and I marveled that his three-hundred-sixty-pound frame (my best guess) fit on that fold-out chair that he brought with him—a reinforced chair, I was hoping, or he was going down with one shift of his ass. You could tell that this man had been a specimen at one time. A mound of muscle, now going to fat. An old forty-something (a lot of best guessing). He wiped a big paw over his face and forced a smile that was not genuine. He sighed like he was about to deliver a eulogy. It was apparent I was just another challenge he had to endure.

He got right into it without a how do you do. "I have to ask," he said in a rich baritone. "What made you think that you were better off dead?" It was the second question he asked. So cut out the bullshit and right to the million-dollar questions. I thought that question was supposed to come up at the end of hours of endless recriminations and breakdowns that led me to consider ending my life crying-towel shit.

He asked my wife if she wanted to stay, and I spoke up. "Not a hope in hell, man," and I realized that I was indeed an asshole. She left without looking back, and I would have done the same. The big man pulled up closer in his protesting-and-stretched-to-the-limit, old-timey bingo chair, putting one thick leg over the other as if he belonged in my hospital room.

"Okay, let's start again. My name's Frank, and I already know yours, so what do you want to talk about?" he asked, less combatively.

"I don't know; how about the price of gas, why cancer is still a thing, and why spinal cord reconstruction hasn't advanced for shit in what, fifty fucking years? But somehow, this is still an exciting time to be a Quad?"

He smiled a bit more, took a deep breath, expanded his massive chest, blew air out slowly, like a tire with a tiny puncture, and looked sad. I didn't know what to make of him. Finally, I decided to cut to the chase. I knew why he was here. "What do I have to do to get out of here? I'm assuming this whole procedure is somewhat scripted."

Now he had a big smile on his face, and he shook his big head, a perfectly round, shaved head. "You're one of those guys, aren't you? The lost dreams and the glory days bullshit. Let me guess, you were heading for the majors or the bigs at one time in your life, now you've lost your mojo and your respect, not just for yourself but for every poor soul that has to endure you?" and he fixed me with the gaze of a man sick of hearing everyone else's lame excuses. The smile was fleeting.

I was stunned into silence. Frank had nailed me right out of the gate. I was so going for bravado, false or otherwise. Now I was just a fish flopping around in a boat. Unsure of my next move, "So . . . like . . . can I go? Or do I have to stay here and listen to you?"

"I don't give a shit, to be honest with you," and he pulled a mound of Kleenex out of the kangaroo pouch of his triple-XL Michigan Wolverines hoodie and snorted like an elephant a few times, checking after every snort to see the results. Finally satisfied, he looked around but couldn't find a garbage can close by, so he stuffed the wad back into his belly pocket.

"That is so fucking gross, man, don't pull that wasted pound of Kleenex out again cause I just might puke."

Now he smiled for real. "Look, partner, you can judge me all you want, but you're the one who tried to pull the plug on life, and I've been here five minutes, I can tell you meant it. Now what? I like my job, but I'm not going to waste my time placating your bruised psyche. It might surprise you to know you're not that original."

"I already have a plan, know where I'm going, and know how to get there," I stated emphatically.

He looked at me, scrutinizing me, shifting around in his protesting little fold-out chair. How that thing maintained its integrity belied reason. He uncrossed his legs and leaned forward over his knees. "Let me tell you how I see it. You feel sorry for yourself because you are not the person you used to be. Surprise, surprise, none of us are. I used to play football. I was a defensive lineman for the Michigan Wolverines. I was all set up with a full scholarship, full fucking ride. I started looking to the big show, the NFL baby, and they were looking at me, the brass ring, welcome to the real bigs, but I blew out my knee in my senior year. It didn't even look like a knee after I was finished with it. Total rebuild, three operations, and months and months of therapy, the knee never did recover, no matter how much I pushed it. I was never the same after that. I'm not saying I can hang with you and we can commiserate together. You're way more fucked up than I ever was, but I know about loss."

"I'll never fucking walk again. I think I've got you crushed for gains and losses, big guy, and I do feel bad about your knee, but I just can't feel for anybody lately, anybody except myself. I am wallowing in self-pity. I've done the fucking steps in my head. Five steps to wellness. Denial, anger, bargaining, depression, and finally, acceptance. It was on a fucking loop. I just crammed another step in-between depression and acceptance, attempted suicide, my step four and a half, and now I'm just getting around to acceptance."

"Are you disappointed it didn't go your way?" He sounded interested for the first time.

"Nope, not anymore. Now I'm just burned out. I've pretty much killed who I was. Now I need time to become this new guy and reinvent myself. I realize that people will have to help me, and I have to let them. That will be the hardest part."

He chuckled, then said, "You're way ahead of the curve. So, I understand you've got a restaurant to run?"

"Not anymore. I'm not going back to that place. It was the beginning of the end, man, and this is the end. Suicide is not even a thought anymore. That thought is riding the rails out of town just like me. I'm going back to the little town where I grew up. It's my Norman Rockwell place."

"I can hold you here, you know? If I wanted to be a prick, you could still be a danger to yourself because I can see from your file that your attempt was quite heroic. You swallowed a bucket-load of drugs and alcohol."

"After all is said and done, do you honestly think having me lay here and stew in my own juices will make me a better person and even more accepting of my condition?"

"Nope, but I'm going to make my buck an hour, so you should listen to me. You're at a point where you have to get selfish."

"Huh?" this was not what I thought I'd hear.

"Selfish. You know, think about yourself. Let me put it this way. You're on the couch, a big comfy couch—in your case a wheelchair—right in front of your T.V., and your favorite team—"

"The Washington Redskins."

"Oh, you poor dumb fuck, no wonder you tried to kill yourself," and a good laugh erupted out of him. A Santa Claus laugh coming out of a big Black dude with a shaved head made me chuckle right along with him. Sure, a little off-color. Maybe Santa Claus was Black after all. How would I know? He continued. "Okay, the Redskins just make me laugh, but let's just say your team scores a touchdown for continuity's sake, and you're stoked, and you want another beer?"

"Okay, you got me. What difference does that make?"

"Keep up. So, you want another beer, and the kitchen is a whole room away, and with the rest of your old buddies sucked up close around the T.V., you have to go through a gauntlet of pissed-off people—because everyone hates the Redskins—to get to the fridge. So *they* would have to get up, move their chairs, whatever, because you're stubborn and want to do it yourself. So you finally get to the kitchen, and now you've got to get the refrigerator door open, you've got to find your preference of beer—"

"Bud Light." I'm warming to his story.

"Oh, you sad fucker. So, you find your Bud Light behind fifteen other assorted beers, and you've got to move them to get to your beer. Then the fridge door gets in your way, and by the time you've quit fucking around, you still have to open the beer can, so you've got to ask someone for help. I have finally arrived at my point. Be fucking selfish. Why not just ask someone to get you a beer in the first place? Why would you miss fifteen minutes of a good football game getting a beer when you could have asked and had an open beer in your hand in thirty seconds?"

"That is one long-ass life lesson, but it makes sense."

"As much sense as cheering for the Redskins."

"Fuck you, I get it already, simple math. If it takes you fifteen minutes and someone else thirty seconds, just ask. It ain't hard to figure out the math on that one." And it continued with more goofy shit that I never thought about.

"Say you drop a coin on the floor. How tough is it to pick it up? Almost impossible for a Quad in a chair, but five seconds for someone else. Just friggin' ask. Most, if not all, people are happy to help. You need to transfer, you've got to go on a commode chair, you can't get your front door open.

Again, just friggin' ask," and he paused and took another deep breath. He was using up all the oxygen in the room.

"Look," he said, surreptitiously glancing at my file. It made me laugh because I really wasn't *that* special. He had probably forgotten my name, but he disabused me of that idea right quick. "So, Mr. Wagner, when I busted up my knee, I was a prick. I had a cane at first. A guy who could wreck a defensive line and sack the living shit out of a quarterback, that guy now has a cane, and my knee is like a live thing pulsing with pain, ready to explode. It was a bitch in line-ups, like bank line-ups, airport ticket line-ups, check outs, you know, where you're waiting forever, and you just ain't moving. So I started packing this chair, this spindly ass chair. It looks like it's going to give out one day, but now I'm going to pack this little fucking thing around until it collapses. So, I'm standing in a line-up with my knee throbbing, it's like a beehive gone crazy right behind the kneecap, and I lean on my chair until I can't stand it anymore. So I unfold it, and I just sit in it, creaking and squeaking, and now that I've taken the time to unfold it, I'm comfortable, and then the line starts moving in front of me. Well, fuck that, the line can just keep moving, and it could get twenty feet in front of me, but I am not folding my chair up because there is still another twenty feet till I'm at the front of the line. Do you get it?"

"Wouldn't someone tell you to get your ass moving and out of your chair?"

"Oh yeah, the odd asshole might say something, and I would just look at him like I would kill him. How many people will ask a ripped, three-hundred-fifty-pound, cranky Black man with a shaved head to pick up his chair and move along? Sometimes I would wait until there was a thirty-foot gap. Do you get my point? Who cares what other people think. Then I would make a big show out of getting up, like every move pained me, and then I would gather up my little chair, fold it nicely, and then stretch. Oh, the stretching part was beautiful. By that time, someone would be saying 'Next, please,' and I would do the thirty feet at my own speed and get my sorry ass to the front of the line."

"Fuck that. I'd have told you to get on with it."

"Okay, I'll give you that cause you seem like a bit of a prick, but very few people would, and you're missing the point."

"Okay, get to the point. Fuck me. Man, oh man, do you tell long stories."

"The point is to *be* fucking selfish. That was an extreme example, but find your limits, your sweet spot. How long will it take me to get a beer? How long will this line-up last? How long until someone gets you a coffee in the morning? And even, how long will it take you to dress? How long to empty your own piss-bag? How long to struggle with a fucking door just to get your sorry ass through it? How long to get a Bud Light out of the fridge? It's all about time management."

"What's that got to do with being an asshole in a wheelchair? If someone gets mad at me, the guys waiting in the line-up, someone who has to put me on a commode chair, they'd just beat my ass, figuratively and maybe literally."

"Yeah, there are some similarities, but some differences too. Mostly, though, I just wanted to tell you my story 'cause it's one of my favorite stories," and with that said, Frank heaved his bulk up to a standing position and then pulled down his pants.

Whoosh, down they went. At least Frank had underwear on, 'cause he dropped 'em right to his ankles. I could see his knee, or what was left of it. It was a lumpy mess, like bruised cottage cheese, exactly where his kneecap was supposed to be, and two ten-to-twelve-inch zippers went down each side of his kneecap. He gave me a healthy viewing, and it would have been a little uncomfortable if someone walked in. Then he pulled up his pants, hitched his belt, and slowly sat back down on his black fold-out chair, with its red nylon seat cover that was squashed all flat and shiny. Then he enjoyed another big sigh and continued. "I suppose I kinda overkilled that, but it means 'find your *own* comfort zone.' What is a specific amount of time for you? It might be a long or a short time for someone else. Whether it's picking up a five-dollar bill in the wind or moving your own ass around in a line-up, it's *your* comfort zone, nobody else's. So, if you have no other choice, get your own goddamned beer. Figure out what makes you happy. If you can't manage that simple thing, you're doomed. You might as well grab a rope and call it a day."

"Man, you suck at being a psychologist or a counselor."

"Oh, Jesus H. Christ, I quit being a counselor five minutes after meeting you. I just didn't feel like moving on. The rest of the day loomed largely, and I wasn't feeling like getting off my ass. It's been a while since I've shown someone my knee, and it felt good. Pretty cool scar, huh?"

"Yeah . . . pretty cool. Good story, nice finish. Um, does this mean we're done? Shouldn't this be *my* show? Do you want to see the scar on my head and neck? Where the fuck are we in this dog and pony show?"

"Oh, you're free to go. Something tells me you'll find your own comfort zone soon enough." He rubbed his big bald head with his catcher's mitt hand, front to back. Then he looked at my hospital bed like he was taking it in for the first time. He finally said, "Yeah, you got that right. I do suck at counseling. I won't tell if you won't, but if you want to talk some more, here's my card. Although I've got a feeling I'm never going to see you again," and he grunted as he got to his feet and almost folded up his little chair. He consciously or unconsciously rubbed his knee, and then Frank plunked right back down, and his tiny chair squeaked in the process, an awful sound like someone strangling a guinea pig. And then we talked for another hour about football, his family and my family, his football choice after college—sure enough, my team's nemesis, the stinkin' Dallas Cowboys. He talked about his rehab and admitted after I questioned him that he had thought about suicide more than once. He called it a knee-jerk reaction. It made him laugh, and he even pulled out that big lump of Kleenex and wiped his nose one more time. It didn't bother me somehow, because it felt like I'd known him for years instead of hours (that makes a big difference in my mind, go figure). He postulated that every person on this Earth has considered or thought about suicide at one time or another. Some more than others.

He finally gave me a pat on my knee, and I didn't feel chided, and I thought, at least someone gets it. "So, this was part of your whole circus act?" I finally asked him.

"Nope," he said, "I just found a kindred soul. You have a borderline Narcissistic Personality Disorder, and you have hurt people in your life. You are manipulative and blame others for your condition, even though you're the dumbass who fell asleep. I could go on, but I don't know you that well. But you did actually *listen* to me, and you showed genuine remorse. So there's hope for you."

"What do you mean, 'borderline narcissistic'? I don't want to be border-line anything."

"Haha, funny guy." And with that, he got up slowly and finally folded up his chair, that fucking thing had to be reinforced, or it should go into a wedding hall museum or something. He gave me a salute, and now that my arms were no longer restrained (he had untied the restraints), I gave back as good as possible. He smiled and said, "Hey, get a dog, and I hope I never see you again." Then he double plunked and one-stepped out of my life.

And he was right. I never saw him again. After that, no one came to visit me except my wife, bless her heart. She told me about the restaurant and how she would make a go of it without me. The staff was doing fine and sent their best.

"Everyone wants to say goodbye," she told me. "So why don't we have a goodbye party?" That was the worst fucking idea I had ever heard. "Oh yeah, and by the way, Bev quit after you ended up in the Psych ward. She'd said you'd understand." Fuck it, I thought. Now that I'm through with the business of dying, let's get on with the business of living.

EPILOGUE

STEP FIVE: UNCONDITIONAL ACCEPTANCE

I WROTE THIS WITH THE knuckle of my right thumb. I'm getting pretty handy at it because I'm sixty-two now. Thirty-two years rushed by like water under a bridge. It's like mercury slipping through my useless fingers. I can look back at that moment in time, and I realize how much life I would have missed if Marie hadn't walked her dog that night and decided she needed a cup of tea.

I've learned a lot. It's simple stuff, really, like if anything takes me thirty minutes to do, and someone assisting me gives up five minutes of their life to help me, then I take the help and smile. Frank was right. If you over-come obstacles, then the people you surround yourself with will do so at the same speed. That and, of course, slow down the line-up, a metaphor that tells everyone to be cool while the rest of the impatient people around you lose their shit.

I've had many home support workers, all so different, with divergent personalities and many quirks to figure out—mine and theirs. I finally made it out of Airdrie two days after Frank released me back to the outside. I loaded up my personal belongings, no old dog, no wagon, and no butter churn. My life fit into one pickup truck. I was now a minimalist. What good were recliners, couches, and chairs to me? I did have five volunteers to drive all the necessary "stuff that worked" back to Maple Ridge. Adams, Rax, Shea, Wok, and Lar, but I only needed one. Funny how shit works out.

I ended up in the Blue Room, an apt nickname for a place to listen and yet be heard. The place I was designated to live in, perhaps from the start. I landed with a thud, and every new experience buoyed me up. Finally, finally, I had arrived, me and my whole Narcissistic Personality Disorder ass. My occupational therapist sister, my younger motherly sister, and my attentive yet still grieving brother (he finally realized he was on his own if he drank too much rye whiskey) were there. Family and parents made my new home accessible, but I made it a home, a place where Randy Wagner lived, and the door was always open. When you worry more about what people think and digest their advice and moods (yes, the people who take care of you have attitudes, too), you become who you are meant to be.

I learned to listen and that grinding your teeth and worrying about all the "shit you can't do" is one big waste of time. It's a new life, and you adapt or die, harsh but true. Home support workers come and go. Some are memorable, like Adrienne, Vicky, Cathy, Joanne, Simran, Shelly, Sally, Evelyn, etc. Vicky, Adrienne, and Cathy became more family than transient helpful paid workers. The list is a lot longer but unnecessary. I salute the people who sign up to help and assist you in finding your own space in the world.

I'm not "cured," for lack of a better word. Sure, I still think about suicide now and then. But, like Frank said, "Don't we all?" The last thirty years weren't better or worse than the first thirty, but they were different. I was different.

I am surrounded and nurtured by family and friends now, and they never gave up on me; they just adapted as I did, and I don't think they even see the wheelchair anymore. They give me a new wheelchair every four or five years—none quite like Bert though. I'm still giving wheelchairs nicknames. I'm at six chairs and counting. Every one of them has its own story to tell. Luckily, I'm still here to tell those stories.

However, one thing that seems worth the telling is why I settled on *Four and a Half Steps* as a working title. Being old gives you hindsight, and if you're lucky like me, you've had the privilege of watching your kids, step kids, nieces, and nephews grow up. I'm so glad I had that experience. They're the ones that come to define me. They got to hear about my "sorry" life, poor little buggers, as I regaled them with stories of my youth. I didn't hold back much with little nuggets of information and indiscretions that might be wise or stupid.

If anyone finds the time to sit down and write, you all have a story to tell. Some stories are sad, some are joyous, and some never get to the starting line. I still don't think suicide is selfish. We've all considered it. One high school friend of mine once said, "It's a good day today. I haven't thought of suicide once," and he's the one that's helping me edit my book, and he hand-painted the book cover. Go figure. I wonder if he thought about his own life while he thought of mine. Like I said, funny how some things work out.

But if you don't have the patience and the foresight to continue, I can't find fault in that because I've been there. So maybe this helps if you're thinking along those lines. Just stop and realize what you might miss and whose lives are bound by yours.

My best advice is to ask for help because you'd be pleasantly surprised at how many people would like that opportunity.

THE END

CPSIA information can be obtained
at www.ICGtesting.com
Printed in the USA
BVHW040253161122
652038BV00006B/45

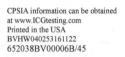